INSPIRATIONAL JOURNAL

"Over 70 special messages to COVID-19 frontliners included from all around the world."

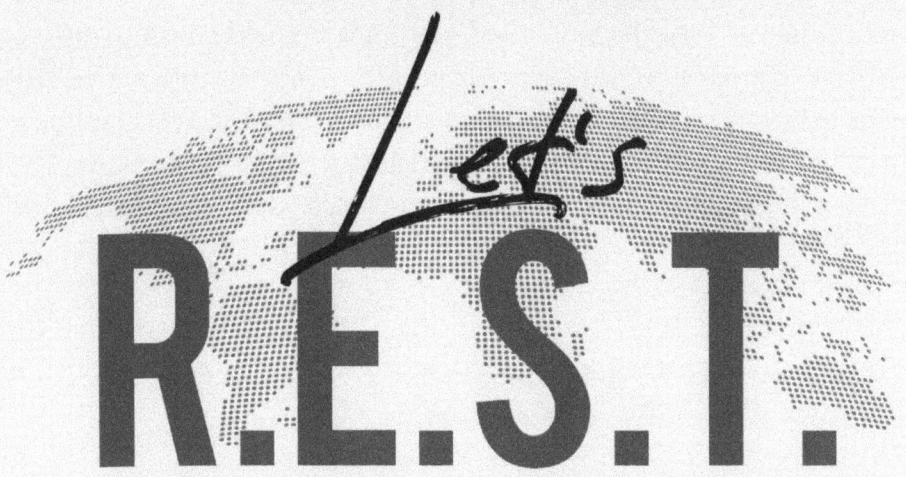

Let's R.E.S.T.
RELEASE EMOTION & STRESS TOGETHER

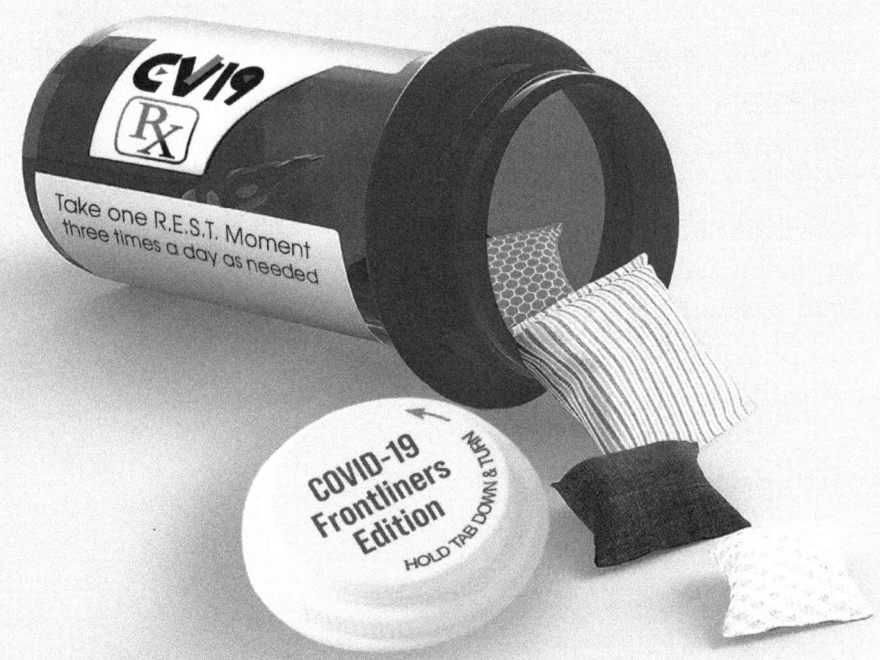

DR. CHEVELTA A. SMITH

Copyright © 2020 Raw Medicine

All rights reserved. No part of this publication may be reproduced, distributed, or transmitted in any form or by any means, including photocopying, recording, or other electronic or mechanical methods, without the prior written permission of the publisher, except in the case of brief quotations embodied in critical reviews and certain other noncommercial uses permitted by copyright law. For permission requests, write to the publisher, addressed "Attention: Permissions Coordinator," at the address below.

ISBN: 978-0-9968295-3-3 (Paperback)
ISBN: 978-0-9968295-2-6 (Hardcover)

Library of Congress Cataloging — Application in Process

Any references to historical events, real people, or real places are used fictitiously. Names, characters, and places are products of the author's imagination.

Front cover image and interior graphic art work by Ikrima Art Studio.
Book design by Raw Medicine/Idea Generator Marketing.
Morning Huddle Music by Epidemic Sound
Editors: Sandra Jones, Ivory S. Bostick, John H. Bostick

Printed by Ingram Sparks, Inc., in the United States of America.

First printing edition 2020.

Raw Medicine
info@drchevelta.com
www.drchevelta.com

Table of Contents

Dedication	1
Foreword	3
Acknowledgements	5
Introduction	7
How To Use This *Let's* R.E.S.T. *Journal*	11
***Let's* R.E.S.T. – It's All About You**	21

Ode to Medical Professionals
Frontliner News
What is Your COVID-19 Story?
How Has the COVID Pandemic Affected You?
Who Were You Before the Pandemic?
How Has the Pandemic Changed You?

***Let's* R.E.S.T.**	35

Release
Emotion
Stress
Together

***Let's* R.E.S.T. – All Around the World**	51

Dr. Chevelta's Morning Huddles for Medical Professionals
Day 1-30

***Let's* R.E.S.T. – More Love From All Around the World**	297
About the Author	313

DEDICATION

First, I would like to dedicate this book to every COVID-19 frontline worker and medical professional throughout the world.

Your hard work and sacrifices have not gone unnoticed. You are impacting lives for the better. You are history makers and are allowing the stories of other people's lives to continue. I am proud of the awesome work you are doing every day.

From one colleague to another, I want you to know that I am praying for you and your families. Moreover, I am specifically praying for your emotional, physical, and spiritual strength to be replenished and sustained during this challenging time in the field of medicine and the world at large.

Together we will get through this pandemic.
I realize that I am not able to be with you physically; however, I want you to know that I am with you in spirit!

I look forward to connecting with you through this *Let's* R.E.S.T. Inspirational Journal.
Even if it's just for a moment, we all need time to Release Emotion and Stress Together.

—Dr. Chevelta A. Smith

FOREWORD

The current COVID pandemic is a huge stressor for medical professionals. Like many of you reading this, Dr. Chevelta is a physician on the frontlines of the fight, who has had her own challenges in life and yet found a way to overcome them. This amazing woman is a board-certified Obstetrician and Gynecologist who served in the Navy and now dedicates her life in service to others. I met Dr. Chevelta long before COVID-19 when I was working at Cleveland Clinic Center for Functional Medicine. We were talking about our own lives - being female physicians, mothers, sisters, daughters, friends, and wives - realizing how day to day stress is the societal norm, and how we are expected to do it all - and do it well. Connecting and commiserating, we knew that being heard, and not being judged, was a part of the healing process. Moreover, we were discussing the negative impact of stress on a person and how it is a cumulative process that impacts our limbic system keeping us in survival mode long term. Even when the stressor is gone, our brain can subconsciously maintain a trauma loop, altering our physiology and brain chemistry leading to an inflammatory state and chronic disease.

As medical professionals, we have the same daily stressors that each human being has, and we also have the additional stress of being frontline responders. Now more than ever, people look to us to protect them and provide them with answers to guide and comfort them. COVID-19 is a virus like no other, and we do not know how to helpfully predict the outcome, give definitive reassurance, or even provide an expected outcome. This is not how we were trained nor how we have experienced medicine; and as a result, this can leave us feeling like we are not rising to the occasion or making a difference.

Some of us approach our daily work with, "it is just another day and I will get through it," or we may find we are not having the empathy for patients as we used to have or dreading going to work. Regardless of our approach, when there is an unknown end or solution, our resilience can wear thin.

Dr. Chevelta has found a way to overcome and thrive. In this journal, she shares her purpose and walks you through each day, providing you with tools to recognize, understand, accept, and release your emotions. She guides you to be your authentic best self and to preserve your emotional capacity for the end of the day to allow you to connect with yourself and your loved ones.

Dr. Chevelta's book reminds you to put YOU first (even for 10 minutes) with self-care and time to have gratitude for the positives in your lives. We have heard it many times, and you probably tell your patients and friends to remember the positive things; but we do not always practice what we preach. We need someone to tell us to stop and focus on the positive of our day and hold us accountable.

This incredible journal is the author's way of speaking to you every day and reminding you to take care of you. As a daily part of your schedule, this journal can impact your performance as a medical professional, friend, colleague, co-worker, parent, child, sibling, spouse, partner, neighbor, and community member. It can improve your sleep, focus, immunity, physical health, and mental well-being. This journal is a collective call for all medical professionals to R.E.S.T.

Dr. Paris Kharbat

ACKNOWLEDGEMENTS

The completion of this journal would not have been possible without the help and support of many. First, I would like to start by giving a HUGE shout out to my dear sister friend (Amy Eversole), sister-in-law (Dr. Cathy Owens-Oliver), and Auntie (Dr. Pat Lewis). Your relentless pursuit in helping me to obtain the wonderful special messages from all around the world for the COVID-19 frontline workers will never be forgotten. Thank you for believing in my vision and responding to my need with much fervor and love. You guys ROCK!

To my birth sisters, thank you so much for your support! Shondale, you have been an amazing teammate on this journey to the completion of this journal. Thank you for your excitement about this project, as well as the countless hours you spent working to ensure its success! Welcome back to the field of Marketing! You did it and I am absolutely honored to be one of your clients. You are talented beyond measure...truly an "idea generator!" To my baby sister, Dr. Shalice McKnight, thank you so much for being a part of this journey. Your feedback and insight as a Psychiatrist was extremely invaluable. Thank you for challenging me throughout this process. I love you dearly!

To my Mom (Pastor Ivory Bostick) and Godmother (Pastor Sandra Jones), thank you for your support in the area of editing! You guys have always been ready and available for every book I've done. Additionally, your encouraging "Mom" words have kept me moving forward and pushing to get this journal done. Thank you for participating in the work of this journal with a desire for its success. I love you two very much. Dad—thank you for believing in me and every book endeavor I have shared with you. Your confidence and trust in my ability to be successful in everything (since I was a little girl) has molded me into the woman I have become today! I appreciate you and love you tremendously! I will always be "daddy's little girl!" To my brother Nate, I love you dearly!

To my beloved family—Smith Crew! (*What it Do?!*). Thank you all for your patience as I worked intently to finish this book. To my husband and my son (Greg & Caleb)—I appreciate your understanding and the sacrifice of precious family time together to allow me to work on this project daily. To my girls (Brooklynn and Morgan Elisabeth)—thank you for cheering me on and affirming me throughout this project. Thank you for loving me and always telling me how "proud" you are of me. It motivated me to keep pushing. I love you dearly!

Finally—I would be remiss not to acknowledge and thank ALL of the contributors to this work. To every individual from all over the world who wrote special messages for this journal—I thank you! From the very beginning, my heart has been overwhelmed by the outpouring of love, appreciation, and honor that you each have shown for the COVID-19 frontline workers and medical professionals who are serving in this 2020 pandemic.

INTRODUCTION

On April 27, 2020, the news announced that Dr. Lorna M. Breen, a well-respected medical director of one of Manhattan, New York's hospital Emergency Departments, committed suicide. She was a COVID-19 survivor and frontline worker. She was a sister, a daughter, and a friend. She was a shero in this war against COVID-19.

I remember reading the article and feeling tremendous sadness. I, too, am a physician, and although I never met her, she was still my fellow colleague. I can only imagine what she may have felt before she left this present world. Medicine, although rewarding, can be quite stressful at times. In fact, the stress amongst all medical professionals has been increasing! We often work long and hard hours while trying to adequately balance between work and home. For some, daily patient loads are becoming greater, while others are overwhelmed with the complexities of their patient's care. The reality: The demands amongst us are significant.

The war against COVID-19 has simply pushed the limit of many medical professionals who were already teetering on the edge of burnout or had actually already crossed over into its territory. This pandemic has added an unforeseen amount of stress upon our medical professionals throughout the world. Not only is it an unfamiliar enemy, in which the common weapons of medical war are ineffective, but it is an invisible enemy that is claiming the lives of its victims at an accelerated rate. Moreover, due to contagiousness, hospitals and medical facilities everywhere have eliminated the ability of individuals to accompany or visit their loved ones in the hospital. As a result, medical professionals have assumed the enormous responsibility to provide a tremendous level of emotional support to their patients who are often critical, lonely, and fearful. Although they give this emotional support willingly, the reality is that it is still very draining and beyond what has ever been expected by our medical providers today. Now, add the constant stress and fear that many medical providers are battling daily regarding the risk to their own lives, and that of their families, each time they return home from a medical facility where known COVID-19 cases are present, or they themselves have been involved in the direct care of those infected. The escalated death rate has turned normal emergency rooms and parking lots into temporary morgues as precious bodies of those succumbing to the virus continue to pile up like casualties on the battlefield. The constant sight of such tragedy, by medical providers everywhere, can be overwhelming. As a result, many have reported sleep disturbances and mood and anxiety changes, which places them at increased risk of developing subsequent mental health disorders that can include trauma and stress-related illnesses. Their minds, although strong, have reached a breaking point. During this time, the desperate need for patient care providers has kidnapped their ability to rest and recover their bodies and minds. The long work hours, lack of sleep, and poor eating habits slowly lead them into a place of burnout and commonly depression. Physicians, nurses, EMTs, medical residents, and medical students are all doing their best to conquer the exhaustion, depression, and daily trauma. However, some have involuntarily surrendered their white flag. In doing so, many have become prisoners of war to depression and traumatic stress, while others, unfortunately, lost their lives to suicide.

In all honesty, the system of medicine will have to change within our society in order for more victories to be won over physician suicide due to burnout. When and if this will occur anytime soon remains to be seen. The death of Dr. Lorna M. Breen, prompted me to think very deeply about what my part could be in helping to alleviate burnout amongst my medical colleagues everywhere during this pandemic. I don't know about you, but I tend to have some of my best think tank sessions in the shower.

One Sunday morning, as hot water beat aggressively on my back, I began to think about a new type of retreat I wanted to launch for physicians to help alleviate the stress we often feel in trying to balance between work and home. I had chosen to name the retreat R.E.S.T. (Release Emotion & Stress Together) because I knew all too well that many of us in the medical profession have difficulty learning how to rest ourselves physically and emotionally. Though I had done some preliminary planning, I put things on pause once national shutdowns and limitations on gatherings due to COVID-19 went into effect.

As I stood in that shower, I heard a still small voice say, "Why wait to launch the R.E.S.T. Physician Retreat. You can help them now." In that moment, I knew God was speaking to me. I realized that I could make an impact in the war against this COVID-19 virus by creating a tool to help medical professionals assess their feelings, emotions, and stress levels in a way that would alert them as to when they were in the danger zone of burnout, stress, and depression. That tool is this *Let's* R.E.S.T. Inspirational Journal!

Why a journal? As medical professionals, I believe we have conditioned ourselves to internalize the stress and anxiety we may feel, because sadly, it is often seen as a sign of weakness when we express that we are overwhelmed, anxious, or depressed. In creating a journal, I wanted to provide a place for frontline workers and all medical professionals now, and after this pandemic, to release stress and emotion together by learning HOW to express feelings, thoughts, and needs.

The ultimate goal of the *Let's* R.E.S.T. Inspirational Journal is to prevent another medical professional from being a causality of burnout, stress, or suicide. If I can help preserve the life of even just one more physician, nurse, resident, medical student, or another colleague, by the simple writing of this book, then I have fulfilled my purpose.

—Dr. Chevelta A. Smith

HOW TO USE THIS JOURNAL

The beginning of the *Let's* R.E.S.T. Journal is created to allow you to express and release your personal feelings, each day, regarding your experience with living in the COVID-19 pandemic. The truth is that as medical professionals, this pandemic has affected us all and tremendously changed our reality. We are no longer practicing medicine in the same manner we did prior to the pandemic, and we will likely never completely return as we develop a new normal. The practice of medicine has not only been changed by the pandemic but so have many of us. As a result, this *Let's* R.E.S.T. Journal provides a space for you to reflect on your experience during the pandemic and *How the Pandemic Has Changed You*—physically, emotionally, and spiritually. There is space for you not only to write what you feel, but also to add photos to capture how the pandemic has impacted you, your family, and the world.

Finally, the second part of our *Let's* R.E.S.T. Journal will serve to walk you through a daily routine of: inspiration, affirmations, self-assessment of your emotions and stress levels, mechanisms to assist you with identifying and coping with your personal stressors, as well as methods to keep you connected together with others.

MORNING:

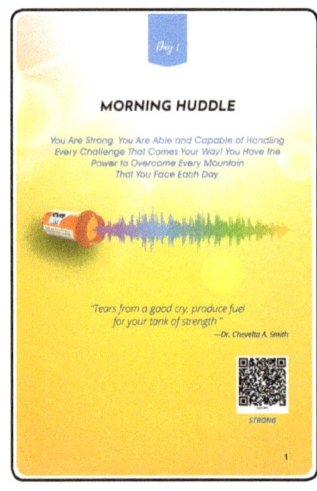

- **MORNING HUDDLE PAGE**

  Enjoy Dr. Chevelta's Morning Huddle for Medical Professionals. These are audio messages full of inspiration, affirmations, and relaxation techniques meant to strengthen your spirit and help you release negative emotions before you start your day. The title of each morning huddle is located underneath the QR code. Additionally, this page also includes a daily quote from Dr. Chevelta, which is often related to the Morning Huddle's focus for the day. As medical professionals working on the same team globally, each huddle serves to connect and rally us together to "conquer" our day! To listen to the Morning Huddles, simply use the camera on your smart phone to scan the QR code at the bottom of the page. If you do not have a phone with this capability, you may visit Dr. Chevelta's website, drchevelta.com, to access the corresponding Morning Huddles each day.

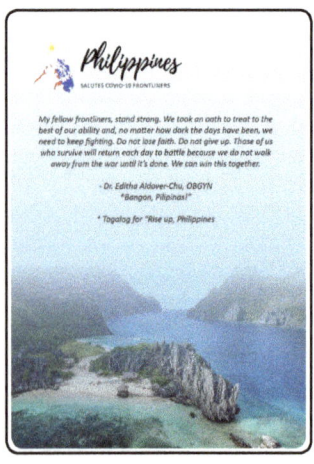

- **TRIBUTE PAGE**

  Following the Morning Huddles, there is a heartfelt message of appreciation written to you, as a COVID-19 frontline worker and medical professional, by individuals representing each of the 50 states and all over the world, including seven continents. These tributes are meant to encourage and uplift your soul.

MID-DAY:

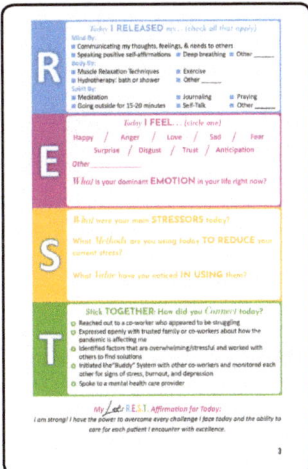

- *Let's* R.E.S.T. ASSESSMENT TOOL™
This is a personal daily assessment chart created to help you Release Emotion and Stress while staying connected with others. An example of the *Let's* R.E.S.T. Assessment Tool is provided at the end of this How to Use This Journal section with instructions on how to use it effectively. This survey will be available daily to help you gauge your emotions and assess how you are handling your stress. It is purposed to be a mid-day check in to assess your mental, physical, and spiritual well-being. At the end of your day, you are encouraged to review your daily *Let's* R.E.S.T. Assessment Tool for completion.

AFTER WORK/PRIOR TO BEDTIME:

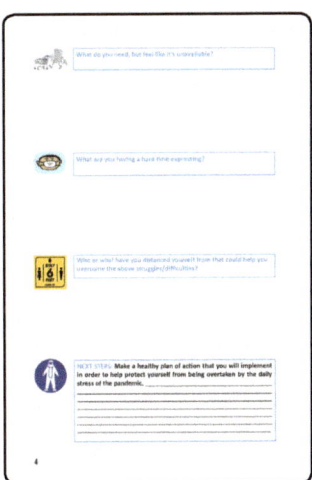

- *Let's* R.E.S.T. REFLECT PAGE
On this page, you will find questions which were created as daily prompts to assist you in releasing various emotions and stressors you may have encountered during the day. This portion of the journal was created to:
  - Help provide an outlet for medical professionals to express deeper personal feelings.
  - Provide a healthy way for medical professionals to cope with the stress they may be feeling both in and out of a pandemic.
  - Build resilience.

- Allow medical professionals the ability to be aware of their current feelings and gauge when and if they are developing unhealthy ways of coping with stress, depression, and/or suicidal ideations.
- Create objective next steps (action plans) for each day that will facilitate stress reduction and/or create an intentional plan towards seeking help from others, including mental health specialists when necessary.

Although it's important to release negative emotions, please be aware that this is also a time to focus on the positive emotions you felt throughout the day. Upon doing so, give yourself permission to outwardly express the joy and happiness you feel when reflecting on those positive emotions. In these instances, the focus should be on releasing the expression of these positive emotions (i.e. dancing around the house like no one is watching, happy shouting, or simply affirming yourself aloud). In addition to releasing negative emotions and stress, this is also a time to "free yourself to celebrate yourself!" You are encouraged to complete these questions at a time when you are relaxed and can focus without interruption.

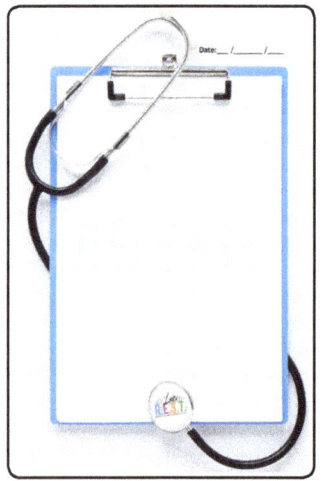

- *Let's* R.E.S.T. RELEASE PAGE
Once you have completed these reflective questions, a blank page has been created for you to write whatever you desire. This is a place for you to release your emotions and stress without prompting. You may choose to write, draw, or doodle. Whatever helps you to release. This is your creative space.

Finally, the last two pages of each day serve to prepare you for your tomorrow and end your day with warmth and appreciation. Here you will find :

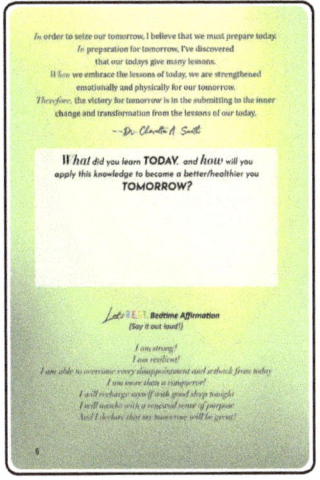

- **TODAY FOR TOMORROW PAGE.** This specific page is designed to help you recognize that each day of life is filled with many "take -aways" or lessons that can empower individuals to become a better version of themselves. Moreover, these lessons can impact how we approach our tomorrows. Once you identify the take aways or lessons learned each day, you will be able to write your individual plan to becoming a better and healthier you!

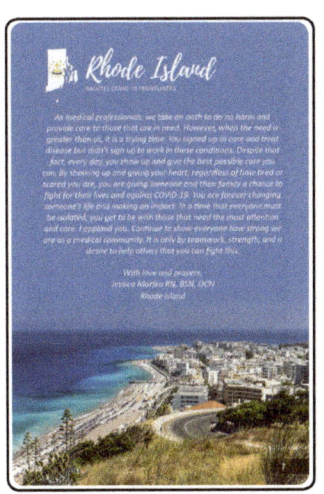

The last page of the day will end with another special message written to you by everyday people who want to remind you that you are appreciated as a frontline worker and medical professional working in this pandemic.

SPECIAL NOTE: Prior to starting your journey through the Let's R.E.S.T. Journal, you are encouraged first to select a trusted person to be your "buddy." Similar to when we utilized the "buddy system" in elementary school to walk the hallways, it is important that you utilize this same system as you walk through the contents of this journal emotionally. Though the purpose of the school "buddy system" has expanded from what it was when I attended elementary school, it was developed to provide a system in which two students would "watch out for each other" and provide emotional support while walking in empty hallways to go to the bathroom, etc. *It could be scary walking through those big hallways as a little person.* The purpose of developing a buddy system with a trusted colleague while using the journal is no different. Your buddy will serve as an individual whom you should commit to staying connected with in order to always have an avenue to express feelings, thoughts, and needs. This should be a mutual relationship in which you each hold one another accountable to truthfully and sincerely express how you are handling stress. Moreover, it is important to communicate when you are struggling to cope in healthy ways and are moving into the danger zone of depression and/or suicidal ideations.

*Let's R.E.S.T.™ is a trademark identity of Dr. Chevelta A. Smith

R

Release: to set free or allow to escape.
Many tend to internalize (hold on) their stress, which over time, becomes detrimental. The purpose of this section is for you to reflect on what specific actions you took that day to help your mind, body, and spirit release stress. The goal is to complete at least one in each category.

E

Emotion: Our state of being.
In this section, you will reflect on how you are currently feeling at that particular moment in time and overall. Honesty and authenticity are encouraged when writing down your emotions.

S

Stress: An emotional factor that creates tension within the physical, spiritual, or emotional states of the body.
In this section, the focus is on stress reduction. Here you will identify specific stressors, express how you are coping with your stress, & indicate the value that these mechanisms are having in restoring your emotional well-being.

T

Together: Jointly, with the unified action of others
This section will reflect how you connected with others (including a Mental Health provider) to implement actions that facilitated the Release of Emotion & Stress personally or in other colleagues & co-workers. I encourage you to develop a Buddy system with a trusted individual and check in with them daily to communicate your needs, thoughts, and feelings. Commit to being vigilant regarding how those working around you may be handling the stress of the pandemic and connect with those that appear to be struggling to assist them with getting help.

DANGER

SELF QUARANTINED

DO NOT ENTER

It is important that you assess your mood daily, in order to recognize when you have moved from the ability to cope with stress in a healthy way and are heading into the **DANGER ZONE** of stress which has the potential to lead to severe depression and ultimately suicide.

When moving into the **DANGER ZONE** of stress the natural inclination is to **ISOLATE** yourself, **QUARANTINE** your feelings, **STOP** talking, & ultimately push others away so that they **DO NOT ENTER** your emotional space!

BE AWARE!!
of self-quarantining feelings of burnout, depression and suicidal ideations!

CONTACT the **National Suicide Prevention Lifeline:** 1-800-273-8255 or **Emergency:** 911
If you feel depressed, suicidal, or just need to talk.

Throughout the *Let's* R.E.S.T. Journal, track your mood and assess whether you are heading into or have entered the DANGER Zone of stress & burnout!

MEDICAL DISCLAIMER

When I decided to write this *Let's* R.E.S.T. Journal, I did so with two goals in mind. The first was my desire to create a tool that could help fellow COVID-19 frontline workers and other medical professional colleagues be aware of when and if they or other co-workers were moving into the danger zone of depression and suicide as a result of the stress from working in this worldwide pandemic. The second goal was to produce a forum/platform in which I could encourage, uplift, and foster connection through inspiration, in an effort to assist in alleviating their daily stress and pressure, if only for a momentary part of the day.

Although I am a physician, I recognize that I am not a mental health specialist. As a result, this journal is not meant to be a medical book. All content found within this *Let's* R.E.S.T. Journal, including text, images, audios, or other formats, were created for informational and inspirational purposes only.

The content is not intended to be a substitute for professional medical advice, assessment, diagnosis, or treatment. Although I am both the author and a board-certified physician, I am not your healthcare provider. As a result, you must always seek the advice of your physician or other qualified health providers with any questions you may have regarding a medical condition. Never disregard professional medical advice or delay in seeking it because of something you have read in this *Let's* R.E.S.T. Journal.

If you think you may have a medical emergency, call your doctor, go to the emergency department, or call 911 immediately.

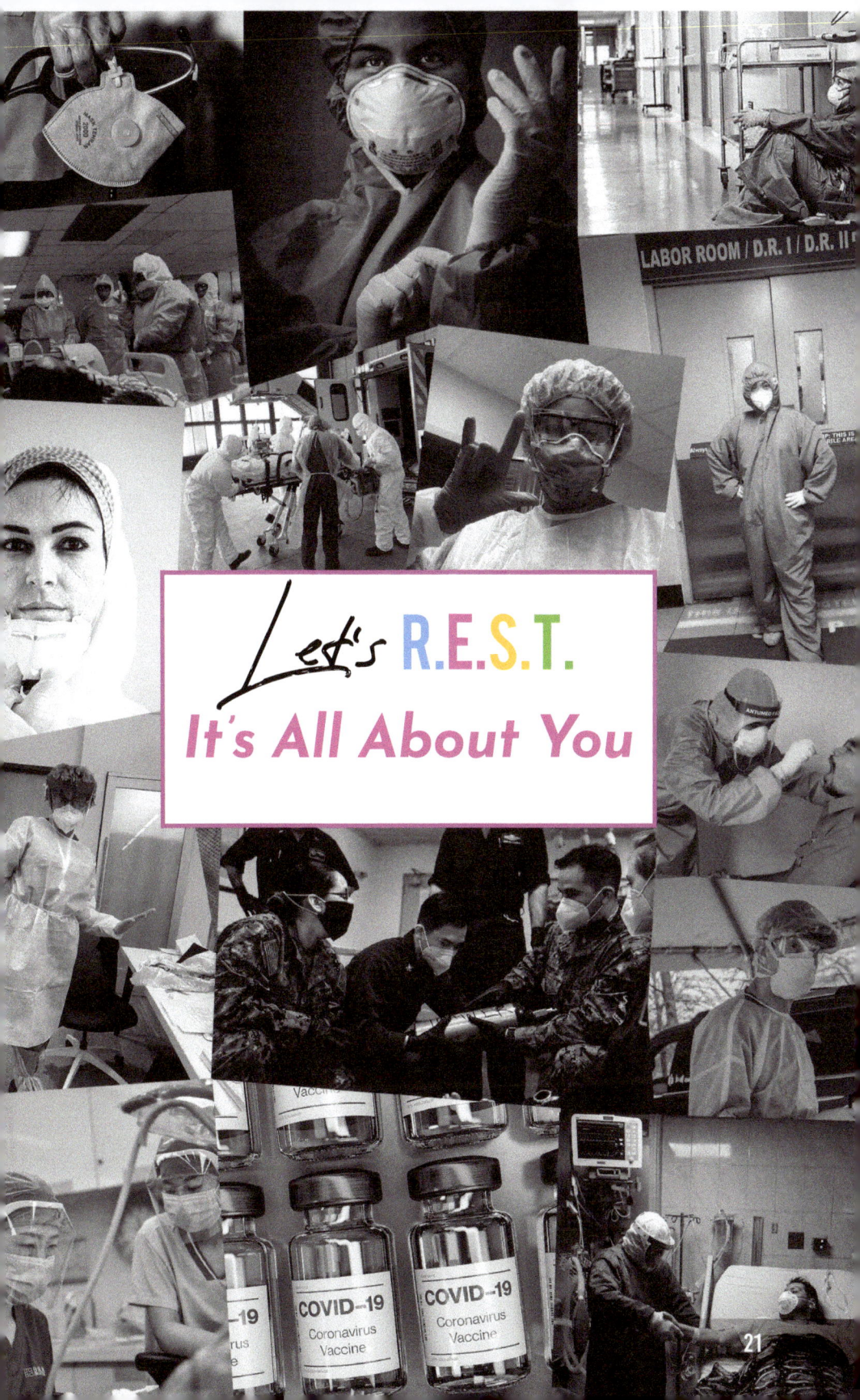

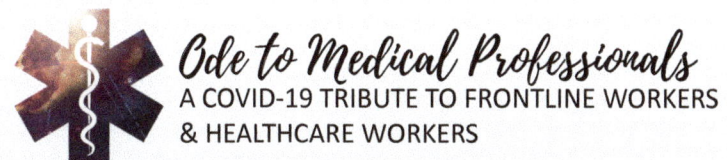

Ode to Medical Professionals
A COVID-19 TRIBUTE TO FRONTLINE WORKERS & HEALTHCARE WORKERS

"I read a book once in 10th grade that led me to describe bone marrow as the vitality of human beings. The heart may receive the most focus, yes, and the face may be granted the most screen time. One's mind does not typically beeline the bone marrow in any case. Yet, here is where the magic happens. Here is where stem cells are produced that can become whatever they want, fortify whichever bodily function they please, as white blood cells, red blood cells, platelets, what have you. You all exemplify biological *magic*. You save lives on regular days while all we encounter from the outside are used scrubs and a tired pair of eyes. You produce life extensions through hard work and dedication so that we can become whatever we want, and so that we can afford to spend our days serving the community in some capacity as well, hopefully transforming our unpayable debt to you into, at the very least, a mutually beneficial relationship.

We, residents of this country, and all those you indirectly save along the way would be nothing without you all. Our frontline medical community: doctors, nurses, technicians, sanitation workers within the field, and everyone in between --- you are the lifeblood, the bone marrow, of this pandemic, just as you are the lifeblood of more "precedented" times. As both of my parents must work outside of the home but are not medical practitioners, I am able to understand just a fragment of your fears and difficulties. I will never fully comprehend the horrors you know and continue to experience. So, I will plead at every intersection that you and your loved ones be met with great health and peace of mind when this period in history comes to a close. But you must know that every life you interact with at work is absorbed into your legacy. Their achievements after recovery are notes on your memoir --- an unending cycle of survival and the beauty formed from your caring, gloved hands."

Daisy O.
Fishkill, New York

07.04.20 / Monday   www.drchevelta.com   Let's R.E.S.T. Journal.

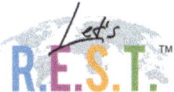 **SPECIAL EDITION** | **COVID-19 FRONTLINE WORKERS** | **STICK TOGETHER** We must be our "Colleague's Keeper"

FRONTLINER NEWS

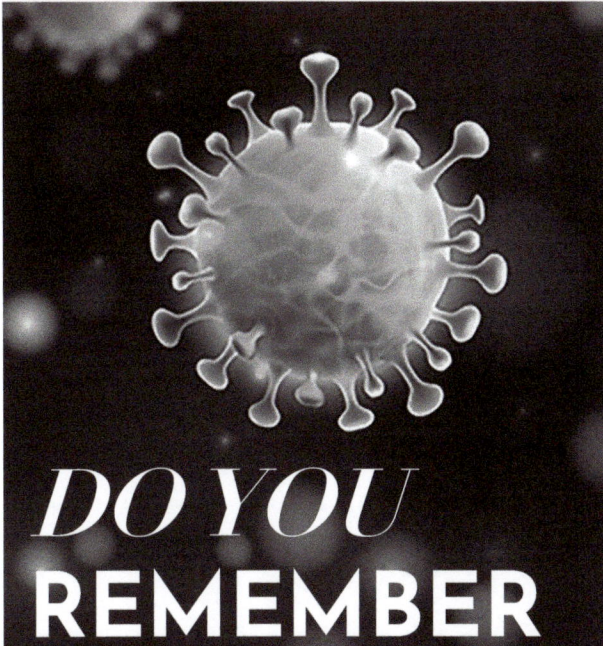

DO YOU REMEMBER

PANDEMIC BEGINS:
Where were you when WHO declared Coronavirus a pandemic on March 11, 2020? *Answer below:*

TOILET PAPER HEIST:
What was the first store you went to only to find no more toilet paper? *Answer below:*

MASK UP:
When did you have to wear your first mask? *Answer below:*

Breaking News

The Coronavirus pandemic has truly transformed the way in which healthcare providers practice medicine and live today.

Who would have ever imagined that we would be required to wear masks outside of the hospital operating room all the time or dress in astronaut looking attire on a daily basis to care for patients? Likewise, did you ever think we'd be stripping down to our skivvies in the garage, upon our arrival home? Who knew that telemedicine visits would one day become the preferred method of providing patient care; elective procedures would be prohibited for a time; and medical professionals everywhere would not only serve as care givers, but also become extended family to the patients they served due to worldwide limitations of who could come into a hospital? When we get through this challenging time, we will have many stories to remember and share.

Continue below ▶

GARAGE STRIPPER:
How did you feel when you had to strip down for the first time, in your garage, before walking into your home after work? *Answer below:*

STAY BACK:
How did you feel when you stood on your first "6 feet apart" floor marker? *Answer below:*

COVID CONTACT:
How did you feel when you had your first known COVID exposure? *Answer below:*

continue to be safe ▶   *continue to stay connected* ▶   *continue to be strong* ▶

25

What is your COVID-19 Story?

How Has the Pandemic *Affected You?*

"Be intentional about assessing your emotional well-being."

Who Were You Before the *Pandemic?*

[Photo of you Here]

> "In keeping connected, it's important that you keep talking."

How Has the Pandemic *Changed You?*

EMOTIONALLY

PHYSICALLY

SPIRITUALLY

Who Do You Want To *Get Back To Being?*

"you have everything in you to recover emotionally and spiritually from this storm called COVID-19."

_____
_____
_____
_____
_____
_____
_____
_____
_____
_____
_____
_____
_____
_____
_____
_____
_____

Create a plan of action to obtain your goal.

_____
_____
_____
_____

" The execution of action is simply the outward manifestation of commitment."

SELF TALK, such as repeating positive affirmations throughout the day, has been shown to reprogram the brain's old beliefs by creating new neuron connections, which then produce new beliefs. These new beliefs ultimately change one's behavior and, thus, their results in life.

Write a personal affirmation that you can repeatedly recite throughout each day as you embark on the journey to restore your emotional well being while utilizing this *Let's* R.E.S.T. Journal

Please see an example below:

I am an excellent...(physician, nurse, etc.)!

I am strong!

I am resilient!

I am important!

I will not be a victim of my stress!

I am emotionally sound!

I am capable of achieving amazing things!

Speak to Yourself!
(Write Your Affirmation Below)

_____
_____
_____
_____
_____
_____
_____
_____
_____
_____
_____
_____
_____
_____
_____
_____
_____
_____

> *Your self-speak and other forms of self-talk are the determining factors in whether the real you, the inside you, wins or loses.*
> —Dr. Shad Helmstetter

Every cloud has a silver lining
John Milton

> **What Positive Impact Has the Pandemic Had in Your Life?**

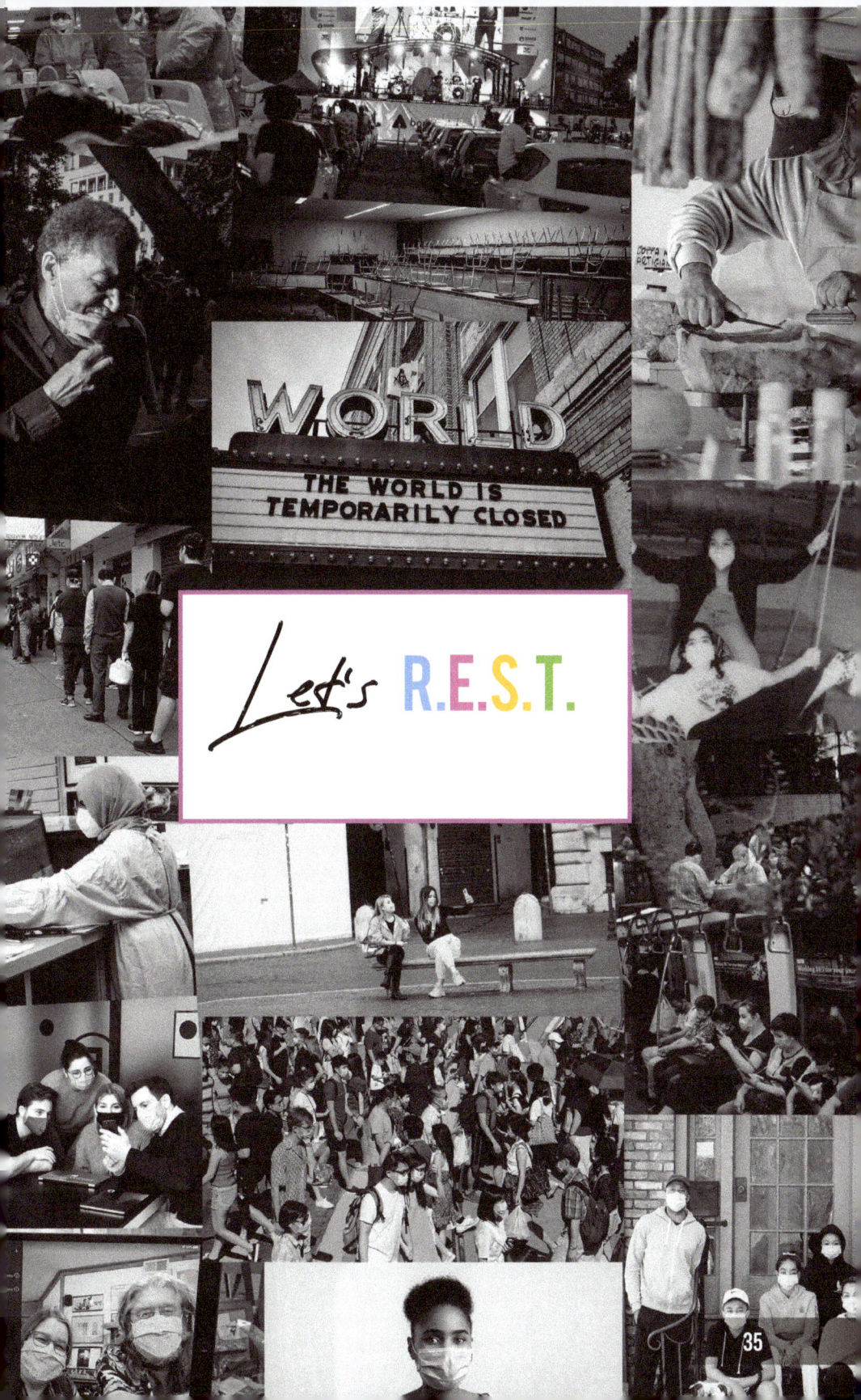

R.E.S.T.

How many times have we heard or said the phrase— "you need to get some rest!" I would bet that we have heard or said it over a million times thus far in our lives. Likewise, how often was it said because either the individual or you yourself were exhibiting behavior consistent with the lack of sleep such as irritability, decreased concentration, inability to think clearly, or just plain zoning out when in conversation with others? The reality is that when those common words "get some rest" are spoken, they commonly refer to the resting of one's physical body. In other words, the hope is that the individual will stop moving so that their body can re-energize and renew its strength. Honestly, we all need rest! Moreover, I believe that we must also remember that the symptoms the physical body often manifests when needing rest is a direct response to what one's soul and spirit are feeling. Therefore, when the mind is overwhelmed and stressed beyond its capability consistently, it can ultimately lead to the development of chronic diseases within the body, including mental illness, which can lead to suicide. Remember, adequate sleep is a wonderful stress reducer, not an eliminator. Moreover, a mind that has not had adequate rest is unable to combat the effects of stress effectively, which can often lead to it being overtaken by burnout, depression, and/or suicide. Thus, there should be a greater emphasis on the need for the mind to rest beyond sleep, but in a way that allows it to Release both Emotion and Stress Together as a community of fellow human beings.

RELEASE

We all have things we need to release emotionally, spiritually, and physically. Honestly, I am not ashamed to say that I have spent most of my adult life figuring out how to do this effectively. You see, I've had many people throughout my life tell me, "you need to let that go" or "get over it," when I'd expressed to them my feelings regarding something or someone that was causing me to feel some level of stress and frustration. Although I totally understand their good intention behind advising me to "let it go," the challenge for me and many others is in discovering how to let it go. It's a phrase we hear often, but rarely does anyone ever explain how to fulfill it. As a result, I spent many years of my life holding onto disappointment, fear, anger, frustration, and sadness, like a toddler clutching her security blanket tightly. It wasn't until my adult years that I realized I was mercilessly dragging my blanket of internalized stress throughout the various years of my life. Unfortunately, there was no security within this blanket, only my personal insecurities, which had changed me over time into someone I had not intended to become. Like every child faced with their parental encouragement to let their security blanket go, I knew that in order to become the person I was purposed to be, I would have to release my insecurity blanket.

Release. I have always felt that to release something truly means that one must first make a conscious decision to do so. In other words, you must be willing to let go. No one else can make that decision for you. It is yours and yours alone to make. This, I believe, is the first step in the process of Releasing. The precursor is that you must acknowledge there are things you need to release. When I make a decision to let something go, I actually say, "I release it" out loud. It's my way of making myself hear those audible words so that my brain can begin the process of rewiring itself. In fact, I want my brain to know that it must reprogram the old thoughts that I developed out of that particular stressful, hurtful, fearful, or disappointing experience. More importantly, I know, as a physician, that thought often dictates behavior. So, like the endless repeating caused by a needle stuck in a record groove, I tell myself over and over again that I choose to release those things and/or people that negatively impact me and my journey to fulfill my God-given purpose. I know that the more my body hears this, it's just a matter of time before my mind believes it. And when my mind believes it, it is just a matter of time before my spirit receives it. Why? Because words are powerful and life changing.

To release something doesn't mean that there is no hurt or pain associated with the decision or the process. I've learned that it is quite the contrary. Sometimes, making the decision to release something or someone can intensify the hurt and pain already in your heart. I believe this to be due to the self-realization that this part of you will never return—at least that's the intent. Remember, if you are like I was, I was great at holding on to feelings for an extremely long time. As a result, they became an inseparable part of me subconsciously and consciously. Therefore, my decision to release things that negatively impacted me still created a void which manifested painful feelings of loss. The reality is that although making the decision to release is a necessary first step, I must then commit to the decision so that I will not regrasp what I purposed to set free so that my healing can begin.

I believe that commitment is not only the second step in releasing but the most essential. Vocabulary.com defines the word commit as "to fully dedicate yourself to something." In learning to embrace all of me and who I am, I learned the importance of "fully dedicating" myself to myself with the intention of becoming the best version of me. In reflecting back over my life, I noted that I was reared to understand the importance of taking care of my siblings as the older sister; as a physician, I was trained to commit myself to the care of my patients; as a wife, I accepted the role to dedicate myself fully to the care of my husband and children; and as a pastor, I promised to dedicate my life to the service of the church, and it's people. Although I remain humble and feel blessed to have had the opportunity to serve in these capacities, I realized that in doing so, I never fully learned how to commit to myself. So, I decided to learn how to do so by taking action.

Once the decision and the commitment to release has been made, then action must be executed. Action is what I believe to be the third and final step in the process of releasing. I believe that the execution of action is simply the outward manifestation of your commitment. I didn't realize this fully until one day when I happened to run across the Merriam Webster definition of commit, which said, "to carry into action deliberately." When I engage in the action of prayer, meditation, and journaling, I am deliberately carrying my decision and commitment to release my spirit. When I engage in the action of positive self-affirmations, deep breathing techniques, and talking to those whom I trust, I am deliberately carrying my decision and commitment to release my mind. When I engage in the action of exercising, muscle relaxation, or simply soaking in a tub, I am deliberately carrying out my commitment to release my body. All these actions I am intentionally engaging in are nothing more than some of the "how tos" for releasing stress, frustration, disappointment, and so on.

What action will you execute to release your stress and anxiety?

EMOTION

Right this moment, my emotions are high. I am angry, sad, and frustrated with the fact that I must accept that the words I typed in this very section—just four days ago—are gone. Yes! My work was on autosave—but it still doesn't change the fact that it is gone now and it can't be recovered. I know this because both my husband and I spent countless hours on the phone with Apple Support and Microsoft Word, as well as massive time on Google and YouTube researching "how to recover the latest version of a Word document." As a grown woman—I sat in my bed, and I cried! My heart sank into a place I had not been in a while. I had spent weeks trying to figure out just how I would write about emotions. I had finally discovered how I would do it, and when I did—it flowed so beautifully. It was something I was proud of. It was something I had accomplished with greatness. Now—it was gone! I had lost it, and both my soul and spirit grieved deeply for the loss I could not recover.

Recover. It hurts when you realize that you cannot regain possession of something lost. Moreover, the intensity of the emotions and feelings that arise in response to your pain feel like a tornado spinning through the territory of your body, soul, and spirit. Like many who have experienced a loss of any kind, I initially refused to let go of the idea that I could not recover what I had lost. I did not want to accept that it was gone forever. If only I could make it come back, I would not have to "do it again and everything would be back to normal." I had allowed my feelings and emotions, arising from this current storm I was in, to cloud my ability to realize that I had everything I needed (strength, courage, resilience) to recover from the wreckage of this situation.
I picked up my inner tools and started to rebuild the words on this page. I recovered.

I have always thought that feelings and emotions were the same. However, it was not until I was preparing to write this journal that I discovered how wrong I was. They are very different and can be complex. One is very evident, while the other can be hidden deep within the depths of one's mind. One is always conscious, while the other is subconscious. . .but can be conscious. One stems from the amygdala, while the other is believed to be neural responses that develop from what's stemming from the unconscious. *Boy, this stuff is confusing. I totally have a new level of admiration for my Neuroscience and Psychology colleagues!*

Simply put, feelings are the conscious physical sensations that manifest when we experience various emotional events (like the butterflies I felt in my gut when I feared I'd forever lost my text). They are always very evident, and we are usually very aware of them. Emotions, on the other hand, are more complex. They often lie within our subconscious mind and reveal themselves only during emotional experiences through our behavior, body language, facial expressions, physiological reactions (increased heart rate), and changes in our voice. Emotions always precede the sensations our bodies manifest as feelings. Although they can be conscious, they can also remain hidden in the depths of our hearts and minds for years until they are discovered. Initially, there was only thought to be six basic emotions (happiness, sadness, fear, disgust, anger, surprise) identified by psychologist Paul Eckman in the 1970s. However, since that time, quite a few more emotions have been recognized. Many believe we develop them through our perceptions and interpretations of specific events based on our culture, upbringing, and direct or indirect experiences. As a result, different people may exhibit a very different emotion to the same exact event.

Honestly, for the purpose of this journal, I don't care if you are able to distinguish between an emotion or feeling. *We can leave that to the experts!* What I do care about is how you are feeling as medical professionals working within a tremendous storm of a pandemic in which there has been tremendous loss and emotional wreckage. I care that this storm, called COVID-19, does not cloud your ability to know that you have everything in you to recover emotionally and spiritually. More importantly, I care that you stay connected to others that can help pull you out from underneath the rubble of despair, depression, guilt, and other emotions that can lead you to the pit of suicide. I created the *Let's* R.E.S.T. Assessment Tool in this journal to help you intentionally assess your emotions. Use it daily. It's important that you recognize when you are no longer handling stress in a healthy way and may be moving into the danger zone of depression and suicide. Be intentional about assessing your emotional well-being and communicating to others when you are not okay. Journaling not only gives you a place to write down what you are feeling but also insight into recognizing your present emotions. Likewise, embrace the positive emotions and feelings you experience each day. Make time to laugh, whether alone (while watching a movie) or in the company of others. The Bible says, "…[It's] good medicine for the soul." Start your day with the Morning Huddles for Medical Professionals. These inspirational messages are meant to add fuel to your emotional and spiritual tanks at a time in our country when they can be depleted quite quickly.

STRESS

I remember, as I'm sure many of my fellow physicians do, sitting in my Anatomy and Physiology class during medical school and learning about the fight or flight response. I was intrigued by what the body could do, especially when it perceived that it was under a particular threat. As my professor reviewed the mechanisms generated by the autonomic nervous system when the body sensed it was in danger, I gained a new appreciation for what I often experienced when I felt stressed and afraid. I now understood that the pounding of my heart against my chest, as well as the increased sweating, sudden ability to move quickly, and the weird twinging sensation I would feel throughout my entire body, were all a part of a wonderful survival mechanism innate to man. Wow. . . The power of adrenaline!

Now, fast forward approximately 25 years later. By some unforeseen turn of events, I unexpectedly found myself sitting in front of my now friend, Dr. Paris Khabart, at the Cleveland Clinic Center for Functional Medicine. As we reviewed the major events of my life, I was surprised that there was even more for me to learn about this widely known "fight or flight" response. I'd always known that the fight or flight response was a cascade event that involved the initiation of stress hormones, which were triggered by a life-threatening situation. However, I always thought that this was only associated with acute life-threatening or sudden stressful events. I had no idea that job stress, marital discord, death of a loved one, and even lifting weights (something I loved to do) were all stressful circumstances that also caused my fight or flight response to be triggered. More surprisingly was the illumination of my understanding that continued (aka chronic) job stress, whether I enjoyed it or not, resulted in the repetitive triggering of this mechanism. Unfortunately, I also discovered that this type of long-term activation would eventually negatively impact the body resulting in such diseases as high blood pressure, insulin resistance, diabetes, obesity, depression, and anxiety—to name a few.

Since I already have a history of hypertension, it was important for me to figure out how to avoid, eliminate, and manage my stress levels.

Stress reduction was my goal. As an OB/Gyn, I knew that my job stress would likely be difficult to change. So, what was a woman with a good amount of type A personality traits suppose to do? Answer: What all of us need to do—avoid and reduce the stress we can control and manage the stress we cannot control. With that said, I started a personal mission to identify the stress in my life and then categorize it as controllable or uncontrollable. The reality is that none of us will ever live a life free of stress. It's impossible and honestly unhealthy. It sounds crazy to say, but there are certain stressors that I've learned to appreciate and welcome. Not because I'm a glutton for punishment, but because I realize that not all stress is bad stress.

It's important to realize that there is healthy stress, which is good, and unhealthy stress, which often has a negative impact on us physically and emotionally. Good stress, "aka Eustress," (like what I felt when working on finishing this book by a deadline)," will often push us to accomplish great things. It makes us better people and heightens our awareness of what we need to do during a specific time frame to stay present on this earth and complete our purpose. Distress, "aka bad stress," like difficult working conditions, creates a constant triggering of the fight or flight response that eventually causes the body to wear down and develop significant health risks. It changes us (our mood and behavior), however, not in a positive way.

So, since stress is here to stay, then we must all decide how to manage it. The steps to doing so are not necessarily difficult but can be challenging. Therefore, it's essential that you're honest with yourself when identifying your stress. As you identify each, write them down. This is why journaling can be quite powerful. It not only provides a place for you to write what you are thinking or feeling but also gives insight into what's stressing you. Once stressors are identified, then I believe the next step is determining whether they're controllable or not. Controllable stressors can be things I commit to doing simply because I didn't know how to say, "no." Controllable stress is what I feel when running late to work because I failed to manage my morning time well when getting ready. These, like other controllable stressors, are things we can reduce or eliminate by simply making better choices.

Uncontrollable stress, like the death of a loved one or loss of a job, are things we cannot control. They're unavoidable; therefore, it's important to learn how to manage them in order to reduce their negative effects on your body.

Learning to manage stress is essential to maintaining homeostasis. Therefore, stress management should always include healthy eating, adequate sleep, and setting boundaries. What will vary amongst each of us is how we choose to do so. You may journal, listen to music, or engage in progressive muscle relaxation. Others may actively exercise, practice deep breathing, or interact with their furry friend. Whatever you do, I believe that a critical step in managing stress is staying connected to others and communicating your feelings and needs with trusted friends, family, and medical providers.

TOGETHER

Community is something we all need as human beings. It's how we identify ourselves, thrive, and survive. In fact— I believe that there is a divine power in the fellowship that community is meant to foster. It is through our fellowship with each other that I believe we learn how to support one another and overcome major challenges. As medical professionals working in a worldwide pandemic, we are currently in a war against an invisible enemy called COVID-19. Similar to any war, I believe that there is power in numbers. As a result, I feel confident that we can and will overcome the physical, emotional, and spiritual toll from this battle if we intentionally remain connected together. By "intentionally," I mean that we are deliberate in maintaining togetherness.

Most people often think of the word "connection" when defining Together. Although I am referring to this common definition when referring to the word, I am also including two of my other favorite definitions—"by combined action and simultaneously" (Merriam Webster). Think about it! If we, as individuals, simultaneously, while in connection with one another, deliberately exerted a combined action of supporting, encouraging, inspiring, and trusting one another, I believe that as frontline workers, this would give many more of us the strength to recover. Although we are being encouraged to socially distance ourselves from each other, I honestly believe that it is our social connection to each other that will be essential to keeping individuals everywhere from becoming emotionally and spiritually depleted. Medical professionals are no exemption. As a result, I hate the term social distancing because what we are actually desiring is physical distancing, which is something very different. Socially, we are not meant to be alone. Alone—in the sense of being isolated. This is why it is imperative that as healthcare providers, we become our "colleague's keeper." Meaning we must keep each other connected to one another. Now don't get me wrong! I realize that we all need "me time." It is these alone moments that often allow us time to process our thoughts, feelings, and emotions. It is also when we often determine how we will handle certain situations and form a plan of action. These times are valuable; however, it is also important that we keep a balance between healthy alone time and crossing the line into isolation resulting from burnout and stress.

In keeping connected, it's important that you KEEP TALKING. This is critical since many individuals can stop talking when they become overwhelmed with stress and anxiety. These harbored emotions and feelings have the potential to lead individuals down the hallway of depression and, for some, through the door of suicide. Therefore, it is important that you stay connected to trusted individuals that have your well-being at heart. As medical professionals, nothing could have ever prepared many of us for what we are seeing and experiencing in this COVID-19 pandemic. As a result, it is not only important that we are staying aware of our emotions and stress, but that we also are communicating to others what we are feeling and need as a result of this overwhelming experience. Honestly speaking, I know that expressing how we feel to others as physicians can be very uncomfortable, especially since medical school and residency unintentionally educated and trained some of us to do the opposite. I say this because, when I was a resident, "suck it up" was the mantra that was repeated like sacred scripture. Unfortunately, for those of us who hid those words in our hearts, we learned to suppress our thoughts, frustrations, and unanswered questions—all for the sake of appearing like a worthy and strong resident. We were afraid of being judged or misinterpreted. Sadly, many of our colleagues, even after completing their training, continue to suppress their feelings, even as veterans in the medical field today. The Good News is that it is not too late to change.

As medical professionals, our resilience is strengthened through the community of togetherness. Therefore, I firmly believe that we must learn to be a safe place for each other to express without judgment. Be approachable and trustworthy. It is in these types of relationships that resilience can be built through authentic communication, collaboration, and shared experiences. I realize that due to our different upbringing, culture, and experiences, we may all handle and communicate adversity and stress very differently. Moreover, I know that it may not feel as natural or comfortable for many of you to communicate how you are feeling. This is why we all must be intentional regarding our commitment to each other and ourselves to remain connected. I can't promise it will be easy, but it is necessary. Utilize the Let's R.E.S.T. Assessment tool to ensure you are intentionally connecting. Keep an eye on each other. Be responsible for your colleague. In other words, look out for their well-being. If he or she appears to be overwhelmed and having difficulty handling stress, don't be silent. I encourage you to reach out to them. You have the right to intrude into their lives under these circumstances. Likewise, don't be offended when a colleague intrudes into your life with caring intent to make sure you are okay. Establish a buddy system with trusted colleagues or friends. The purpose of this relationship is to hold each other accountable in the area of communicating your feelings on a daily basis. If a few days have gone by and you have not heard from your buddy—call or text them to make sure they are okay. If, for some reason, you do not feel comfortable sharing your feelings with a friend or colleague, then at least communicate with your health care provider where you are emotionally. We have all gotten to where we are through the help of others. Don't stop now. Togetherness is key.

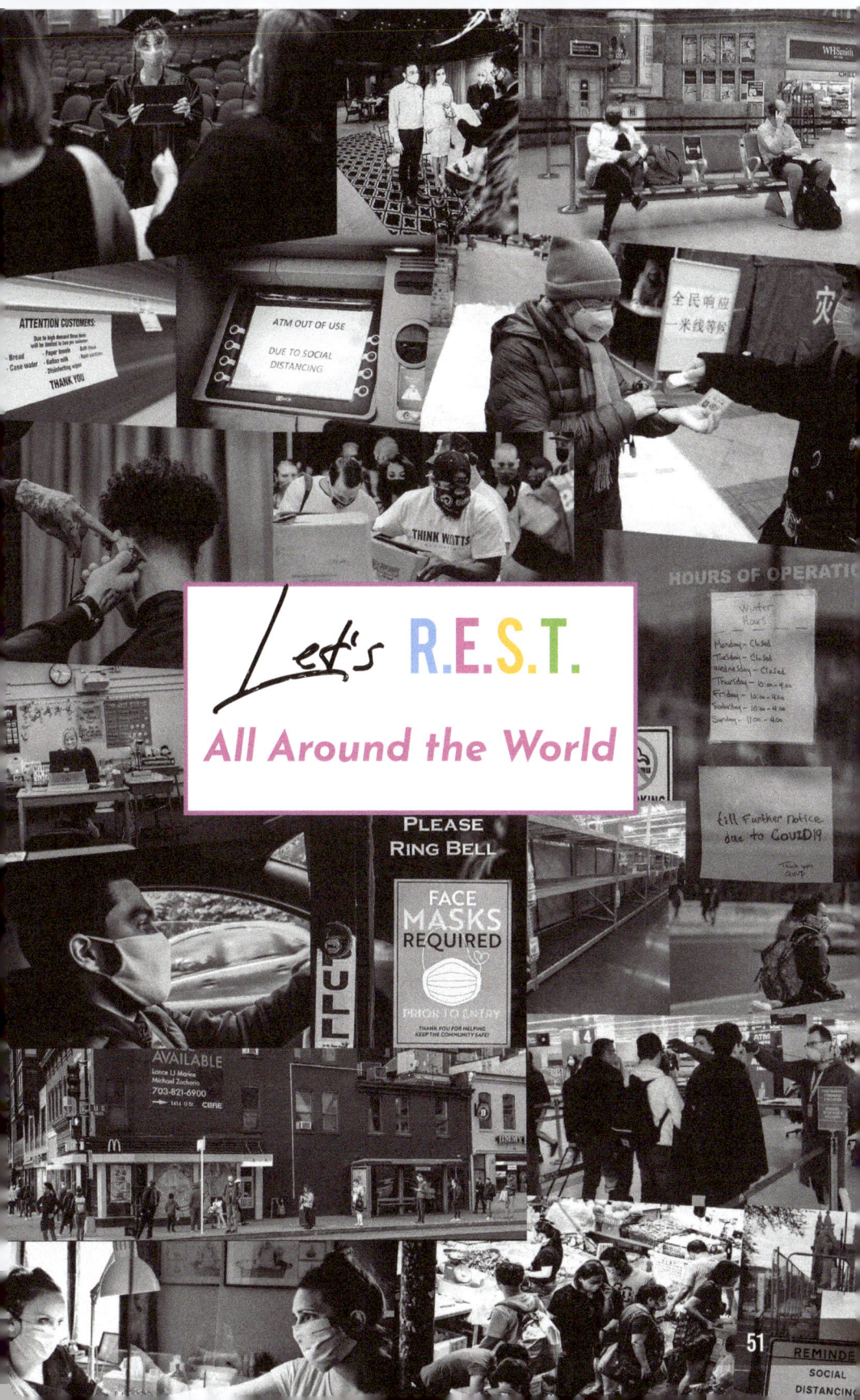

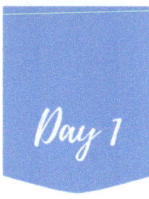

Day 1

MORNING HUDDLE

You Are Strong. You Are Able and Capable of Handling Every Challenge That Comes Your Way! You Have the Power to Overcome Every Mountain That You Face Each Day.

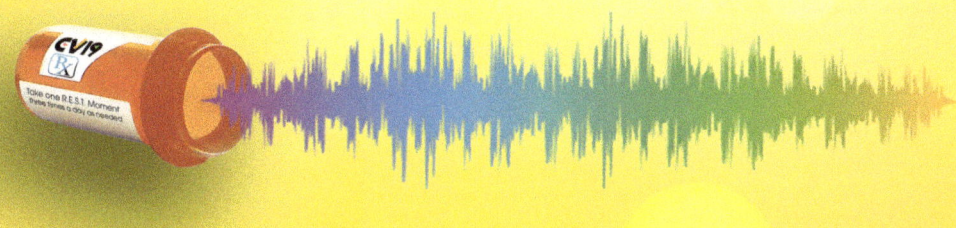

"Tears from a good cry, produce fuel for your tank of strength"

—Dr. Chevelta A. Smith

STRONG

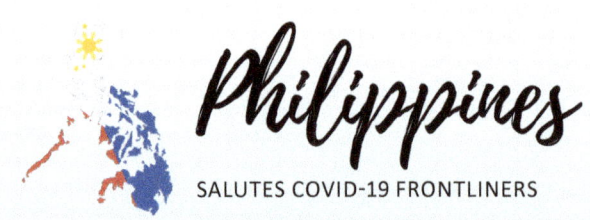

Philippines
SALUTES COVID-19 FRONTLINERS

My fellow frontliners, stand strong. We took an oath to treat to the best of our ability and, no matter how dark the days have been, we need to keep fighting. Do not lose faith. Do not give up. Those of us who survive will return each day to battle because we do not walk away from the war until it's done. We can win this together.

—Dr. Editha Aldover-Chu, OBGYN
*"Bangon, Pilipinas!"

* Tagalog for "Rise up, Philippines"

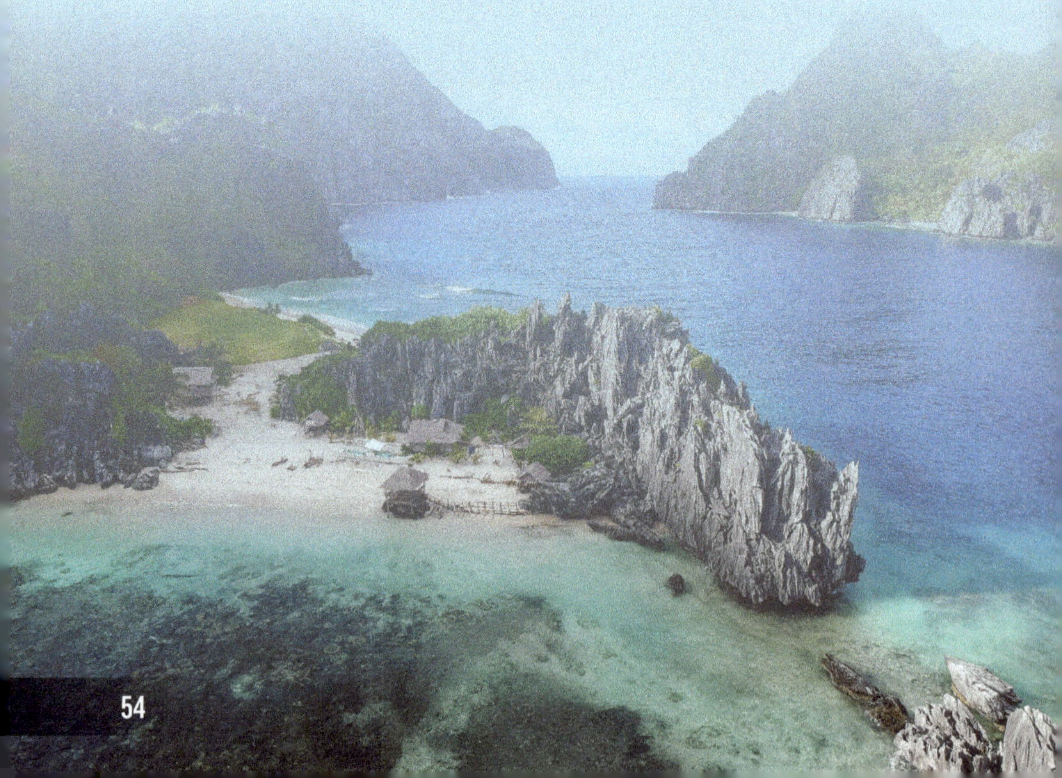

R — Today I RELEASED my... (check all that apply)

Mind By:
- Communicating my thoughts, feelings, & needs to others
- Speaking positive self-affirmations
- Deep breathing
- Other _____

Body By:
- Muscle Relaxation Techniques
- Exercise
- Hydrotherapy: bath or shower
- Other _____

Spirit By:
- Meditation
- Journaling
- Praying
- Going outside for 15-20 minutes
- Self-Talk
- Other _____

E — Today I FEEL... (circle one)

Happy / Anger / Love / Sad / Fear

Surprise / Disgust / Trust / Anticipation

Other _____

What is your dominant **EMOTION** in your life right now?

S

What were your main **STRESSORS** today?

What *Methods* are you using today **TO REDUCE** your current stress?

What *Value* have you noticed **IN USING** them?

T — Stick TOGETHER: How did you *Connect* today?

- Reached out to a co-worker who appeared to be struggling
- Expressed openly with trusted family or co-workers about how the pandemic is affecting me
- Identified factors that are overwhelming/stressful and worked with others to find solutions
- Initiated the "Buddy" System with other co-workers and monitored each other for signs of stress, burnout, and depression
- Spoke to a mental health care provider

My *Let's* R.E.S.T. Affirmation for Today:

I am strong! I have the power to overcome every challenge I face today and the ability to care for each patient I encounter with excellence.

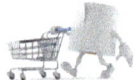
What do you need, but feel like it's unavailable?

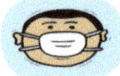
What are you having a hard time expressing?

Who or what have you distanced yourself from that could help you overcome the above struggles/difficulties?

NEXT STEPS: Make a healthy plan of action that you will implement in order to help protect yourself from being overtaken by the daily stress of the pandemic. _____
_____
_____
_____
_____
_____
_____

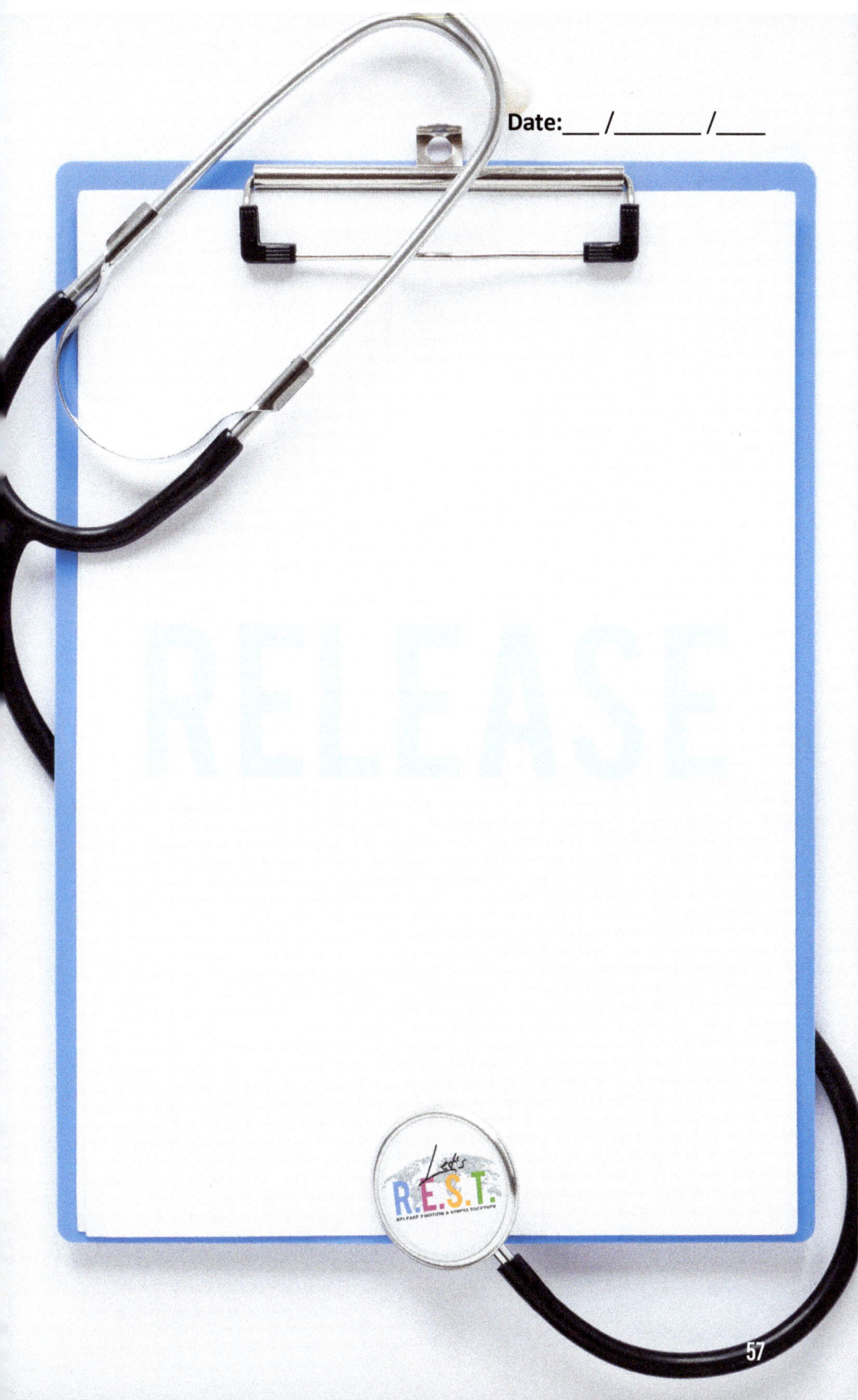

In order to seize our tomorrow, I believe that we must prepare today.
In preparation for tomorrow, I've discovered
that our todays give many lessons.
When we embrace the lessons of today, we are strengthened
emotionally and physically for our tomorrow.
Therefore, the victory for tomorrow is in the submitting to the
inner change and transformation from the lessons of our today.

—— *Dr. Chevelta A. Smith*

What did you learn **TODAY**, and *how* will you apply this knowledge to become a better/healthier you **TOMORROW?**

Let's R.E.S.T. Bedtime Affirmation
(Say it out loud!)

I am strong!
I am resilient!
I am able to overcome every disappointment and setback from today
I am more than a conqueror!
I will recharge myself with good sleep tonight
I will awake with a renewed sense of purpose
And I declare that my tomorrow will be great!

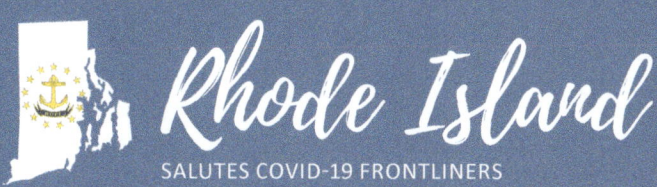

Rhode Island
SALUTES COVID-19 FRONTLINERS

As medical professionals, we take an oath to do no harm and provide care to those that are in need. However, when the need is greater than us, it is a trying time. You signed up to care and treat disease but didn't sign up to work in these conditions. Despite that fact, every day, you show up and give the best possible care you can. By showing up and giving your heart, regardless of how tired or scared you are, you are giving someone and their family a chance to fight for their lives and against COVID-19. You are forever changing someone's life and making an impact. In a time that everyone must be isolated, you get to be with those that need the most attention and care. I applaud you. Continue to show everyone how strong we are as a medical community. It is only by teamwork, strength, and a desire to help others that you can fight this.

With love and prayers,
—Jessica Marfeo RN, BSN, OCN
Rhode Island

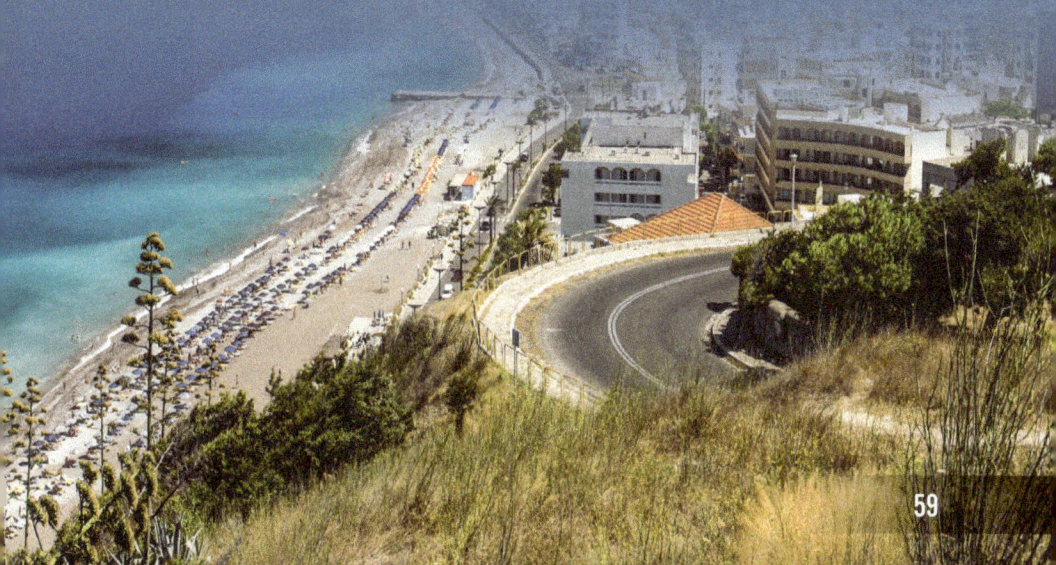

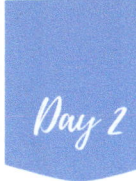

MORNING HUDDLE

Equip Yourself in a Way That Will Keep You Emotionally and Spiritually Protected. Equip Yourself With Peace, Joy, Love, and Courage.

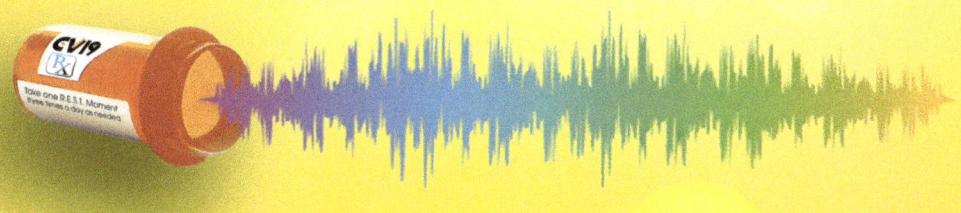

"Victory comes when your mind won't let anything else in."

—Dr. Chevelta A. Smith

EQUIP

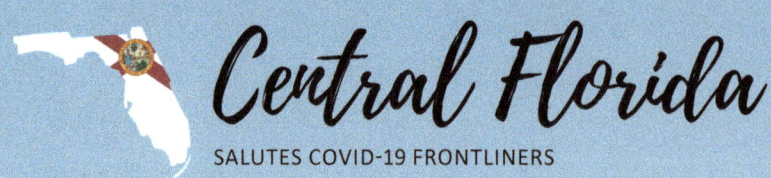

Central Florida
SALUTES COVID-19 FRONTLINERS

When I was a child, I watched TV and read about superheroes that would scoop in and save the day, but they were just fictional characters. Today, our hospitals and healthcare facilities are filled with real women and real men who dress in PPE to save the lives of people across this country. Thank you to the healthcare workers who put their lives on the frontlines in the battle against COVID-19. You are the real deal!

—V. Fleming
Central Florida

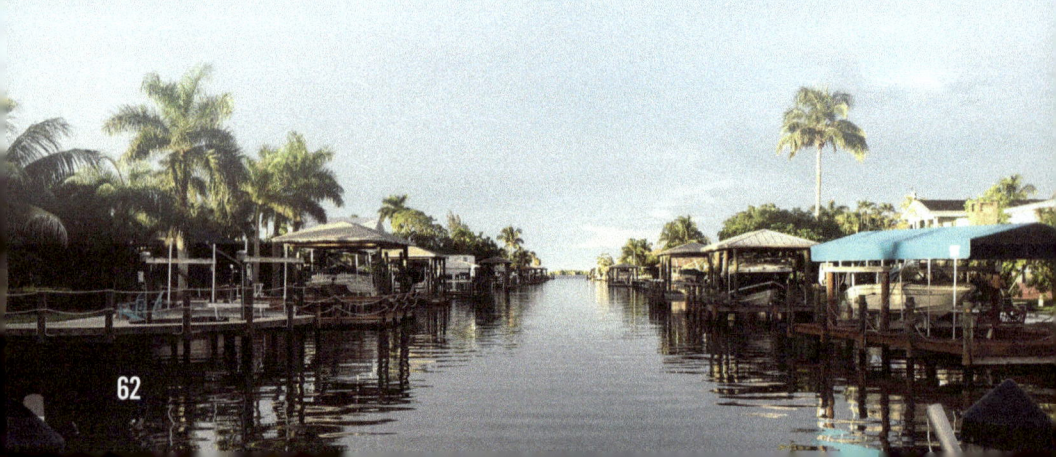

R

Today I RELEASED my... (check all that apply)

Mind By:
- Communicating my thoughts, feelings, & needs to others
- Speaking positive self-affirmations
- Deep breathing
- Other _____

Body By:
- Muscle Relaxation Techniques
- Exercise
- Hydrotherapy: bath or shower
- Other _____

Spirit By:
- Meditation
- Journaling
- Praying
- Going outside for 15-20 minutes
- Self-Talk
- Other _____

E

Today I FEEL... (circle one)

Happy / Anger / Love / Sad / Fear

Surprise / Disgust / Trust / Anticipation

Other _____

What is your dominant EMOTION in your life right now?

S

What were your main STRESSORS today?

What *Methods* are you using today TO REDUCE your current stress?

What *Value* have you noticed IN USING them?

T

Stick TOGETHER: How did you *Connect* today?

- Reached out to a co-worker who appeared to be struggling
- Expressed openly with trusted family or co-workers about how the pandemic is affecting me
- Identified factors that are overwhelming/stressful and worked with others to find solutions
- Initiated the "Buddy" System with other co-workers and monitored each other for signs of stress, burnout, and depression
- Spoke to a mental health care provider

My *Let's* R.E.S.T. Affirmation for Today:

I am equipped with everything I need to fulfill my purpose today in the lives of my patients, co-workers, and family.

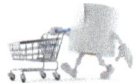
What do you need, but feel like it's unavailable?

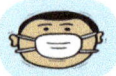
What are you having a hard time expressing?

Who or what have you distanced yourself from that could help you overcome the above struggles/difficulties?

NEXT STEPS: Make a healthy plan of action that you will implement in order to help protect yourself from being overtaken by the daily stress of the pandemic. _____
_____
_____
_____
_____
_____
_____

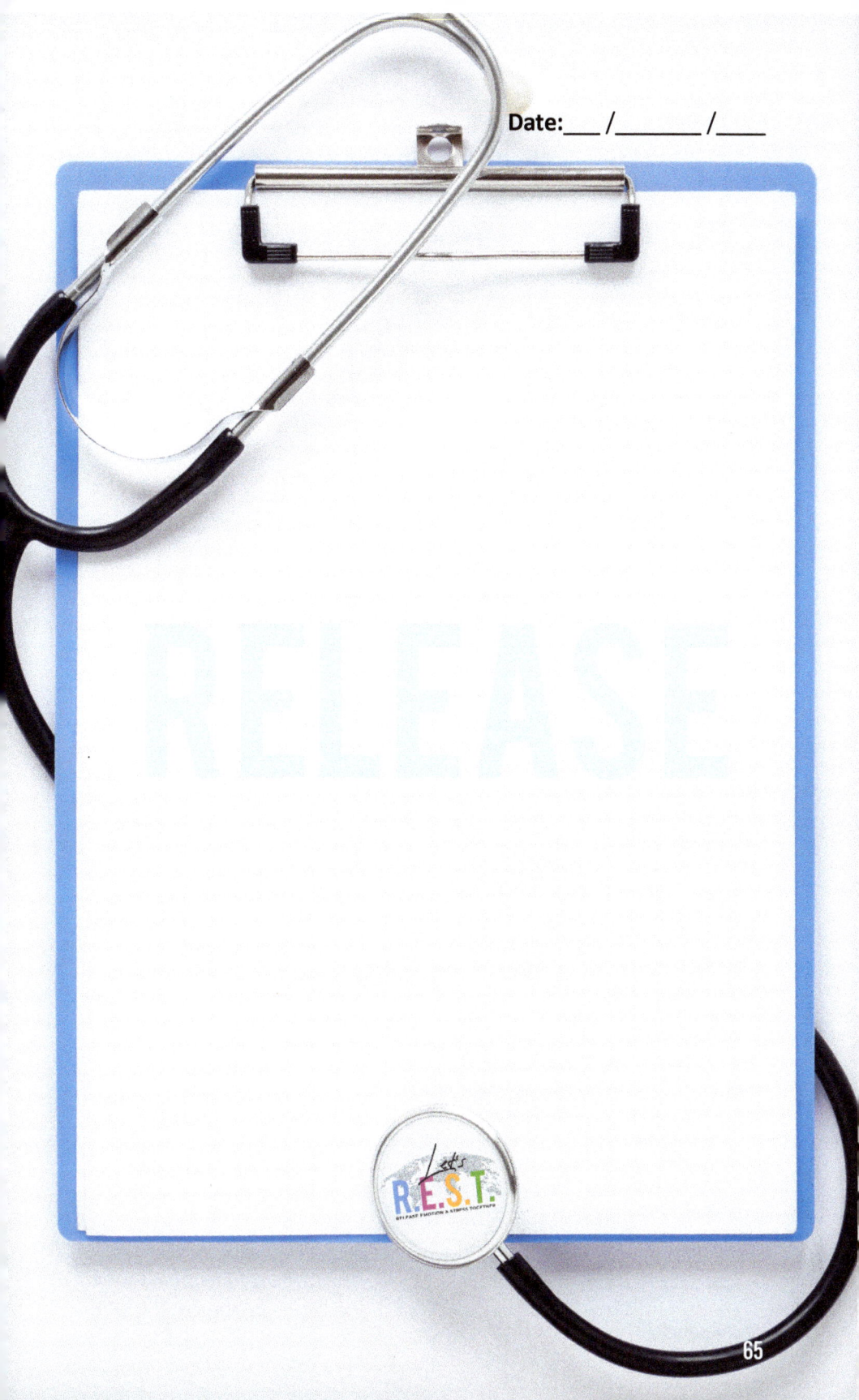

Date:___ /_____ /____

RELEASE

In order to seize our tomorrow, I believe that we must prepare today.
In preparation for tomorrow, I've discovered
that our todays give many lessons.
When we embrace the lessons of today, we are strengthened
emotionally and physically for our tomorrow.
Therefore, the victory for tomorrow is in the submitting to the
inner change and transformation from the lessons of our today.

--Dr. Chevelta A. Smith

What did you learn **TODAY,** and *how* will you apply this knowledge to become a better/healthier you **TOMORROW?**

Let's R.E.S.T. **Bedtime Affirmation**
(Say it out loud!)

I am strong!
I am resilient!
I am able to overcome every disappointment and setback from today
I am more than a conqueror!
I will recharge myself with good sleep tonight
I will awake with a renewed sense of purpose
And I declare that my tomorrow will be great!

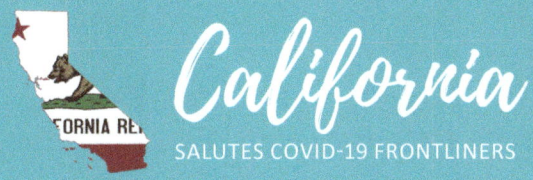

California
SALUTES COVID-19 FRONTLINERS

We are here for a divine purpose. I know the road has been tiring and scary, but everything we are doing is not in vain.
We have been given the opportunity to care for those who are facing a crippling infection. We have been able to deliver compassion because we, too, are fighting this virus. Thank you for all you've done and are doing. Thank you for being the real-life Superman and Superwoman. The world is indebted to you.

—G.Askia
Elk Grove, California

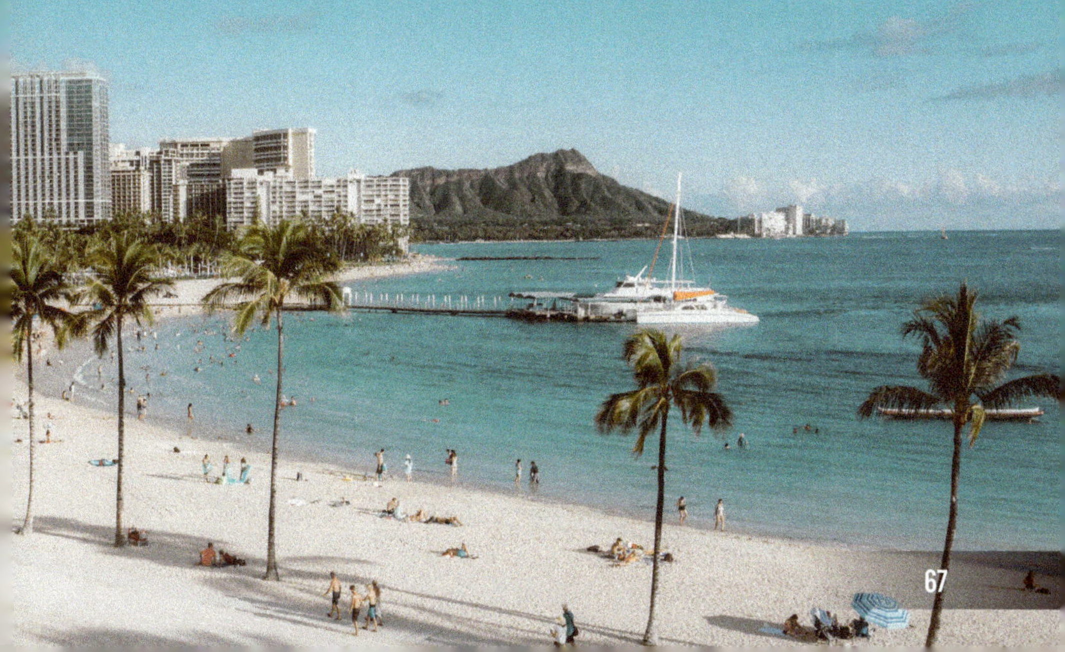

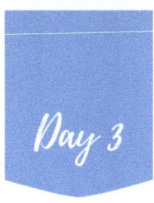

Day 3

MORNING HUDDLE

It Is So Important That We Make Time Throughout Our Day to Release Negative Emotions and Stress.

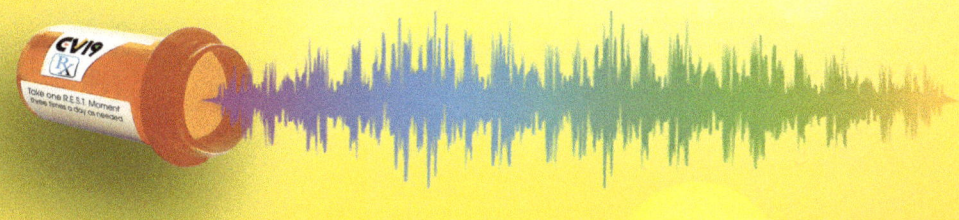

"Silence!—I'm renewing my mind."
—Dr. Chevelta A. Smith

PAUSE

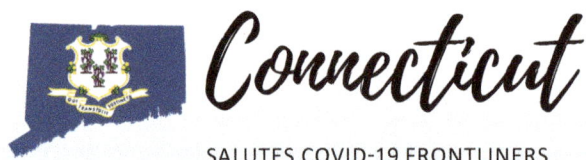

Connecticut

SALUTES COVID-19 FRONTLINERS

Give yourself a break. Mourn the losses but celebrate the wins with fervent joy. Don't forget that you are being prayed for by thousands of people every day whose inherent hope is for you to be successful in the treatment of this illness. You are not forgotten. You are loved and appreciated. Keep fighting this horrific beast of a virus, and we will continue to cheer you on in your diligent endeavor.

—Amy E.
Torrenton, Connecticut

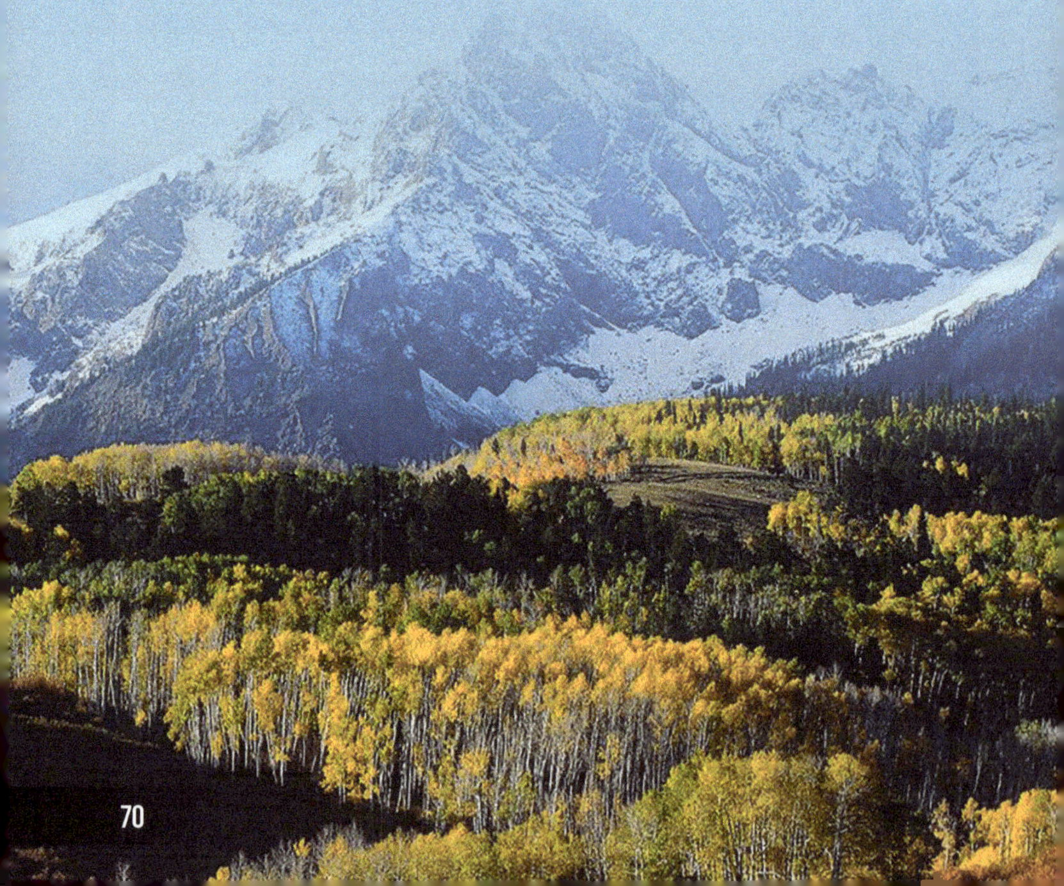

R

Today I RELEASED my... (check all that apply)

Mind By:
- ■ Communicating my thoughts, feelings, & needs to others
- ■ Speaking positive self-affirmations ■ Deep breathing ■ Other _____

Body By:
- ■ Muscle Relaxation Techniques ■ Exercise
- ■ Hydrotherapy: bath or shower ■ Other _____

Spirit By:
- ■ Meditation ■ Journaling ■ Praying
- ■ Going outside for 15-20 minutes ■ Self-Talk ■ Other _____

E

Today I FEEL... (circle one)

Happy / Anger / Love / Sad / Fear

Surprise / Disgust / Trust / Anticipation

Other _____

What is your dominant **EMOTION** in your life right now?

S

What were your main **STRESSORS** today?

What *Methods* are you using today **TO REDUCE** your current stress?

What *Value* have you noticed **IN USING** them?

T

Stick TOGETHER: How did you *Connect* today?

- ○ Reached out to a co-worker who appeared to be struggling
- ○ Expressed openly with trusted family or co-workers about how the pandemic is affecting me
- ○ Identified factors that are overwhelming/stressful and worked with others to find solutions
- ○ Initiated the "Buddy" System with other co-workers and monitored each other for signs of stress, burnout, and depression
- ○ Spoke to a mental health care provider

My *Led's* R.E.S.T. *Affirmation for Today:*
I will take a pause whenever I feel overwhelmed. I will restore my strength. I will thrive.

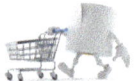 What do you need, but feel like it's unavailable?

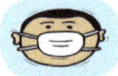 What are you having a hard time expressing?

 Who or what have you distanced yourself from that could help you overcome the above struggles/difficulties?

 **NEXT STEPS:** Make a healthy plan of action that you will implement in order to help protect yourself from being overtaken by the daily stress of the pandemic. _____
_____
_____
_____
_____
_____
_____

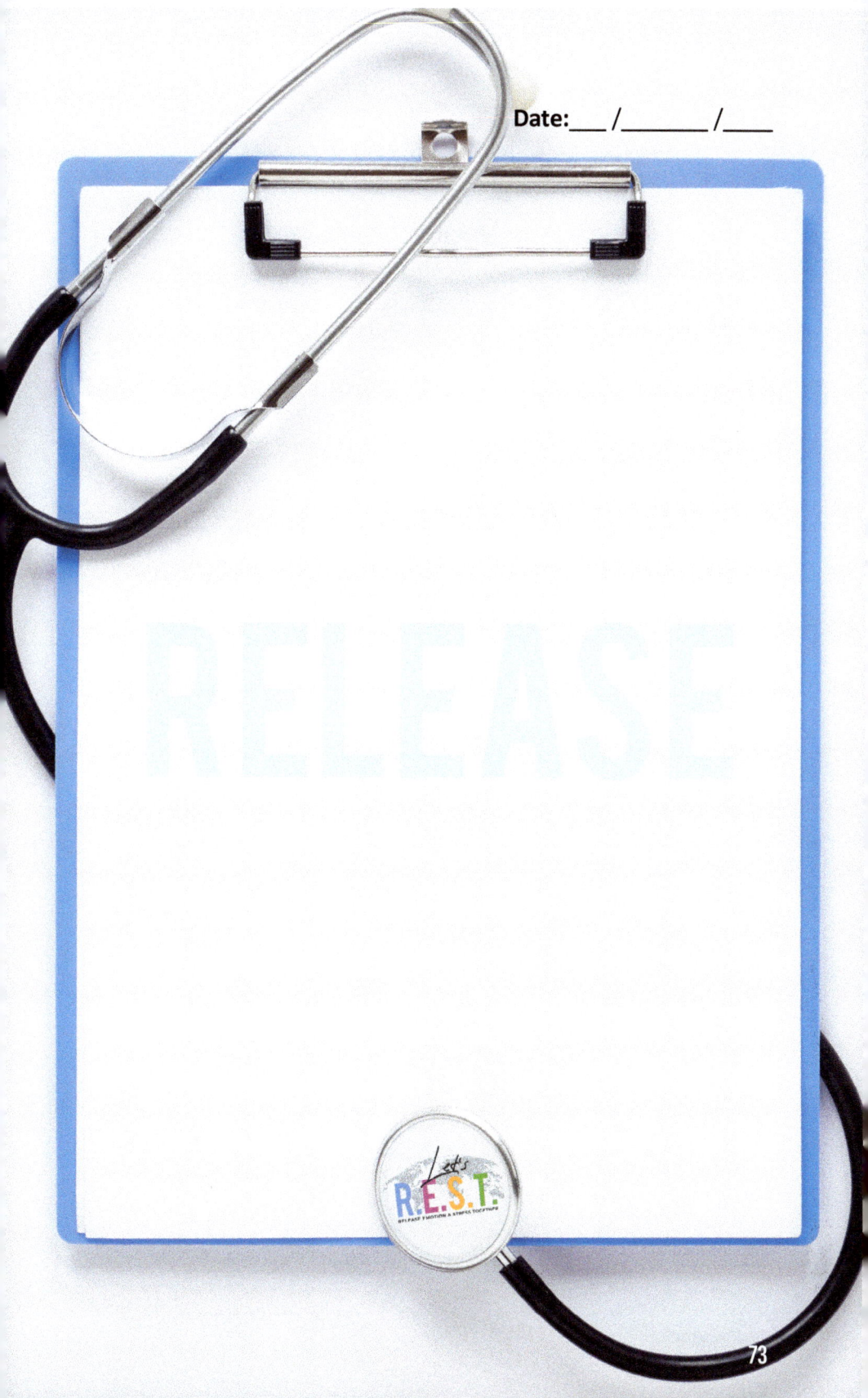

In order to seize our tomorrow, I believe that we must prepare today.
In preparation for tomorrow, I've discovered
that our todays give many lessons.
When we embrace the lessons of today, we are strengthened
emotionally and physically for our tomorrow.
Therefore, the victory for tomorrow is in the submitting to the
inner change and transformation from the lessons of our today.

--Dr. Chevelta A. Smith

What did you learn **TODAY,** and *how* will you apply this knowledge to become a better/healthier you **TOMORROW?**

Let's R.E.S.T. **Bedtime Affirmation**
(Say it out loud!)

I am strong!
I am resilient!
I am able to overcome every disappointment and setback from today
I am more than a conqueror!
I will recharge myself with good sleep tonight
I will awake with a renewed sense of purpose
And I declare that my tomorrow will be great!

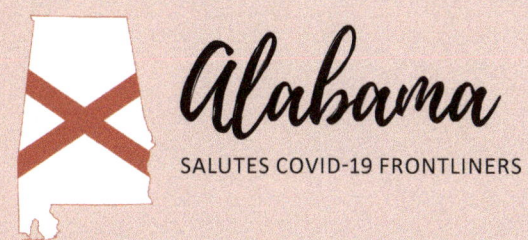

Alabama
SALUTES COVID-19 FRONTLINERS

I serve as a pastor for a local church in the fine city of Enterprise, Alabama. I have two sisters who are nurses. When they share with me how hectic it is for them, as they fulfill their oath to serve others through their profession; it reminds me of the hymn written by Ruth Cave Jones, which says,

In times like these you need a Savior,
In times like these you need an anchor;
Be very sure, be very sure,
Your anchor holds and grips the Solid Rock!

Doctors and frontline workers, the men and women that are working tirelessly to keep our loved ones safe, are the epitome of this monumental hymn. They are our anchor to normalcy. They are our savior from the Coronavirus. I thank God that their anchor holds and grips the solid rock to give of themselves and to help those that have succumbed to the vestiges of this pandemic. I thank my Lord and Savior for them.

God bless you greatly,

—H. G. Rogers
Enterprise, Alabama

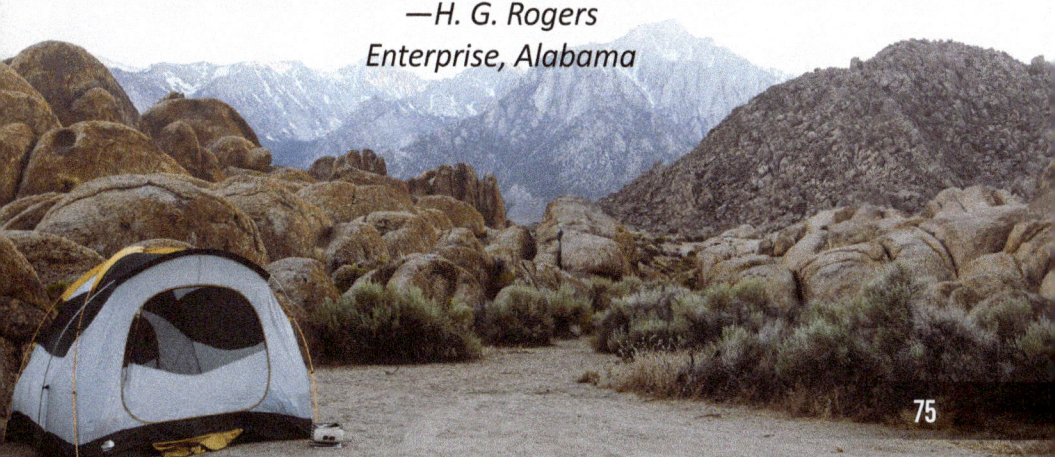

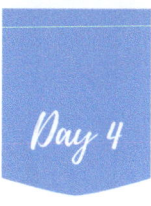

Day 4

MORNING HUDDLE

Commit to Living a Happy Life. Let Go of Unforgiveness. Let Go of Disappointment. Let Go of Your Pain and
Live a Happy Life Ever After.

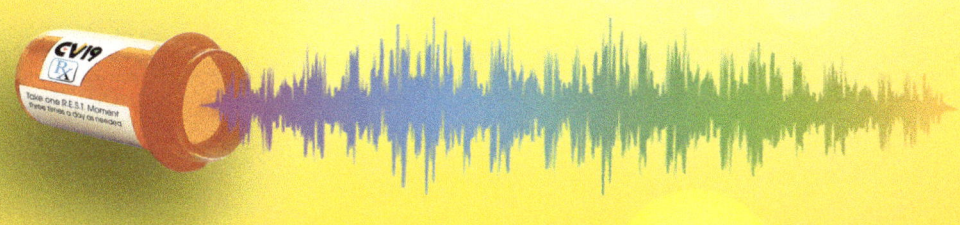

"Rewrite the narrative of your life with a theme of happiness."

—Dr. Chevelta A. Smith

AFFIRMATION HAPPINESS

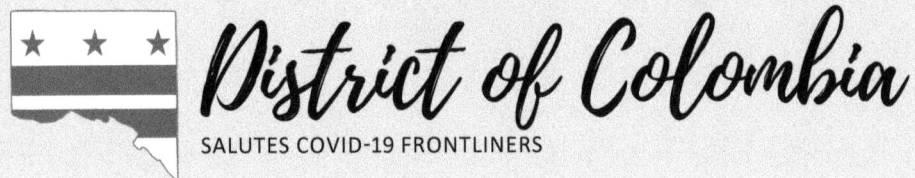

District of Colombia
SALUTES COVID-19 FRONTLINERS

To all of The Frontline Workers of COVID-19, no matter what the situation may look like, keep the joy of the Lord in your heart and in your mind. You were specially chosen to help bring health and life to those in need. Don't Give Up Now! We need you in order to defeat COVID-19!

Sending Love, Support, and Prayers from Washington, DC!

—Jackie B. and MiKayla B.
District of Columbia

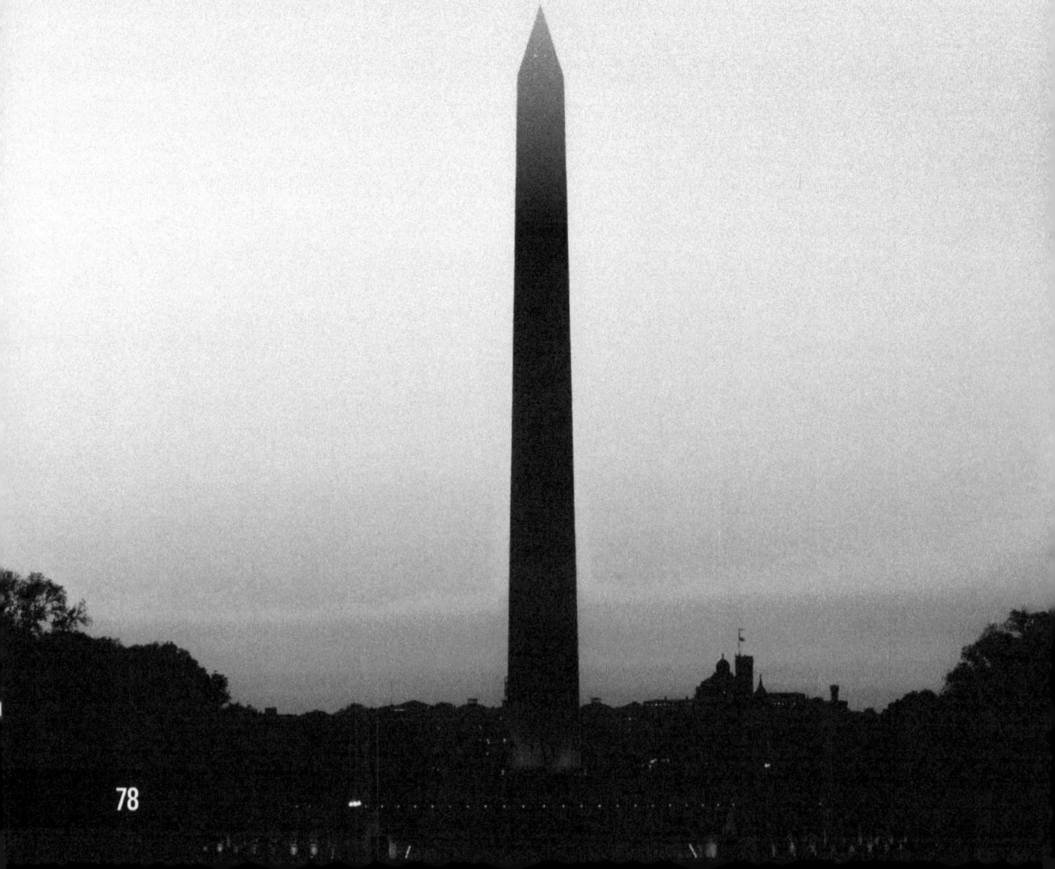

R

Today **I RELEASED** *my*... *(check all that apply)*

Mind By:
- Communicating my thoughts, feelings, & needs to others
- Speaking positive self-affirmations ■ Deep breathing ■ Other _____

Body By:
- Muscle Relaxation Techniques ■ Exercise
- Hydrotherapy: bath or shower ■ Other _____

Spirit By:
- Meditation ■ Journaling ■ Praying
- Going outside for 15-20 minutes ■ Self-Talk ■ Other _____

E

Today **I FEEL**... *(circle one)*

Happy / Anger / Love / Sad / Fear

Surprise / Disgust / Trust / Anticipation

Other _____

What is your dominant **EMOTION** in your life right now?

S

What were your main **STRESSORS** today?

What *Methods* are you using today **TO REDUCE** your current stress?

What *Value* have you noticed **IN USING** them?

T

Stick TOGETHER: How did you *Connect* today?

- Reached out to a co-worker who appeared to be struggling
- Expressed openly with trusted family or co-workers about how the pandemic is affecting me
- Identified factors that are overwhelming/stressful and worked with others to find solutions
- Initiated the "Buddy" System with other co-workers and monitored each other for signs of stress, burnout, and depression
- Spoke to a mental health care provider

My *Let's* **R.E.S.T.** *Affirmation for Today:*
I choose to be happy! I deserve to be happy! I am happy.

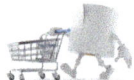

What do you need, but feel like it's unavailable?

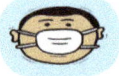

What are you having a hard time expressing?

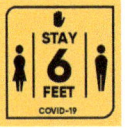

Who or what have you distanced yourself from that could help you overcome the above struggles/difficulties?

NEXT STEPS: Make a healthy plan of action that you will implement in order to help protect yourself from being overtaken by the daily stress of the pandemic. _____
_____
_____
_____
_____
_____
_____

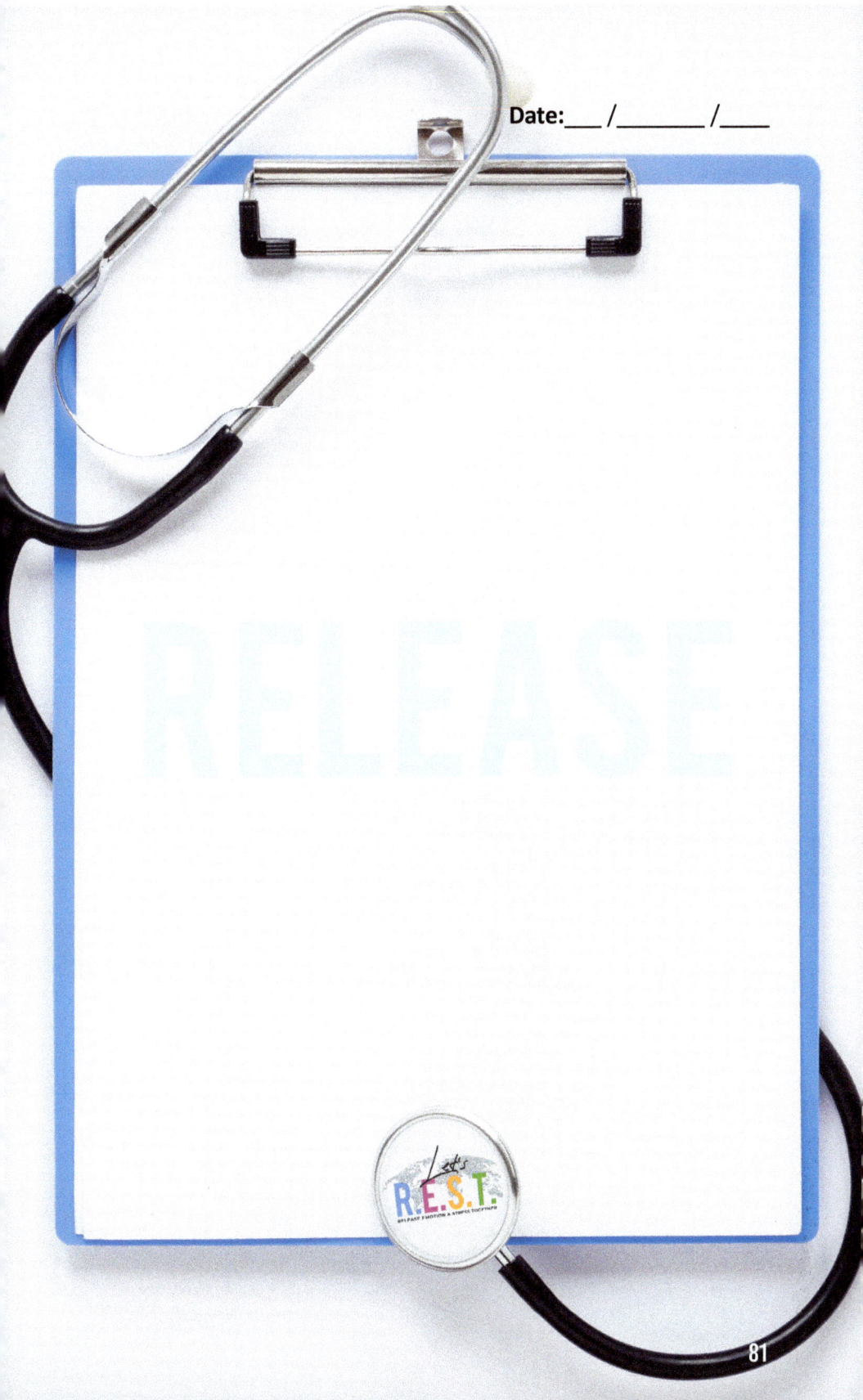

Date:___ /_____ /___

RELEASE

In order to seize our tomorrow, I believe that we must prepare today.
In preparation for tomorrow, I've discovered
that our todays give many lessons.
When we embrace the lessons of today, we are strengthened
emotionally and physically for our tomorrow.
Therefore, the victory for tomorrow is in the submitting to the
inner change and transformation from the lessons of our today.

—— Dr. Chevelta A. Smith

What did you learn **TODAY**, and *how* will you apply this knowledge to become a better/healthier you **TOMORROW?**

Let's R.E.S.T. **Bedtime Affirmation**
(Say it out loud!)

I am strong!
I am resilient!
I am able to overcome every disappointment and setback from today
I am more than a conqueror!
I will recharge myself with good sleep tonight
I will awake with a renewed sense of purpose
And I declare that my tomorrow will be great!

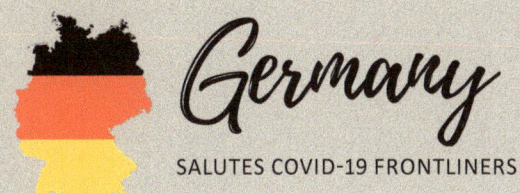

Germany
SALUTES COVID-19 FRONTLINERS

Ihrseid die Helden des Alltags. Die Menschen mit dem Herz am richtigen Fleck. EureLeistung und Hingabe in dieserherausfordernden Zeit istunbezahlbar. KämpftweiterihrHelden. Wirsind in GedankenbeiEuch und dankenEuch von ganzem Herzen. Bleibtgesund! GottesSegen

(English Translation):
You are the heroes of everyday life -- the people with their hearts in the right place. Your performance and dedication in this challenging time are priceless. Keep fighting you heroes. We are with you, in our hearts, and thank you from the bottom of our hearts. Stay healthy and blessed.

—Jessica I.
Germany

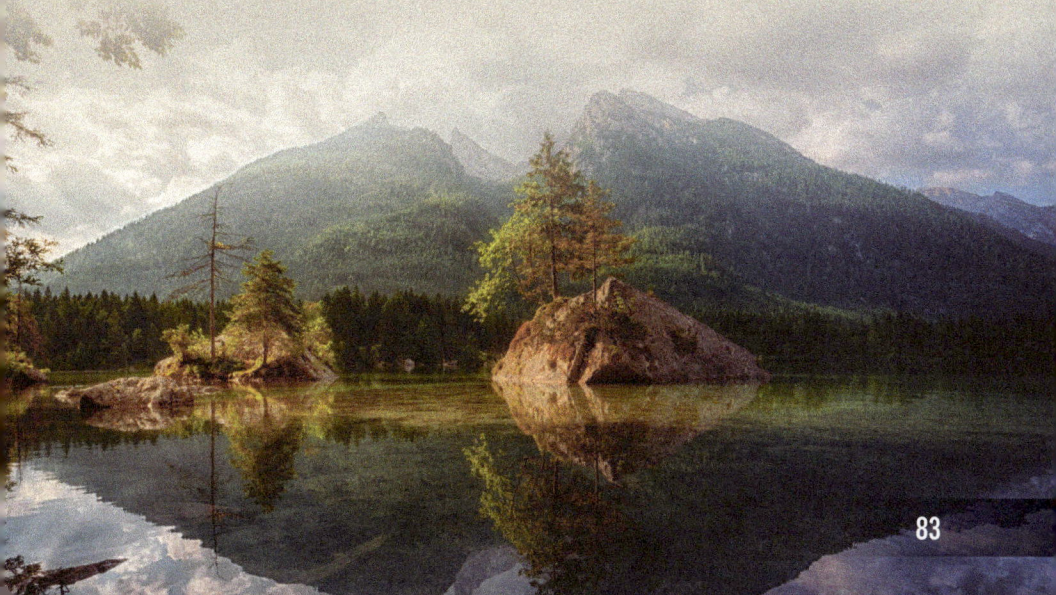

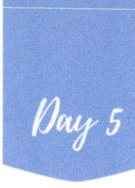

Day 5

MORNING HUDDLE

You Are Full of Multiple Talents, Different Skills, and Different Assets. Stir Up Those Gifts That Are Within You. Rekindle Your Passions and Your Dreams.

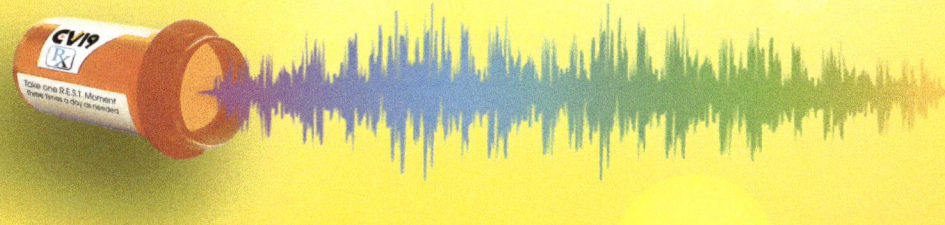

"Don't limit yourself to only moving and functioning in one aspect of who you are."

—Dr. Chevelta A. Smith

STIR UP

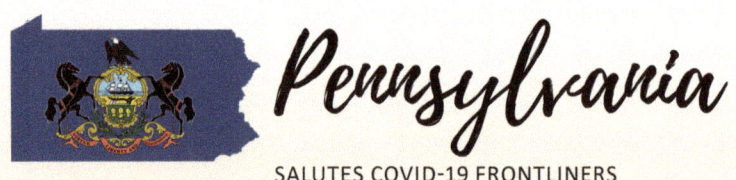

Pennsylvania

SALUTES COVID-19 FRONTLINERS

Thank you from the bottom of our hearts for being the light in this darkness. Your skill, compassion, and selflessness are saving everyone you touch, even those who pass to their next life. Your strength and commitment are saving us all. Take good care of yourselves and know that the whole world is watching and carrying you through this. We are forever grateful for your presence at this moment!

All our love,
—Kathy, Mark, and Zoe D.
Pittsburgh, Pennsylvania

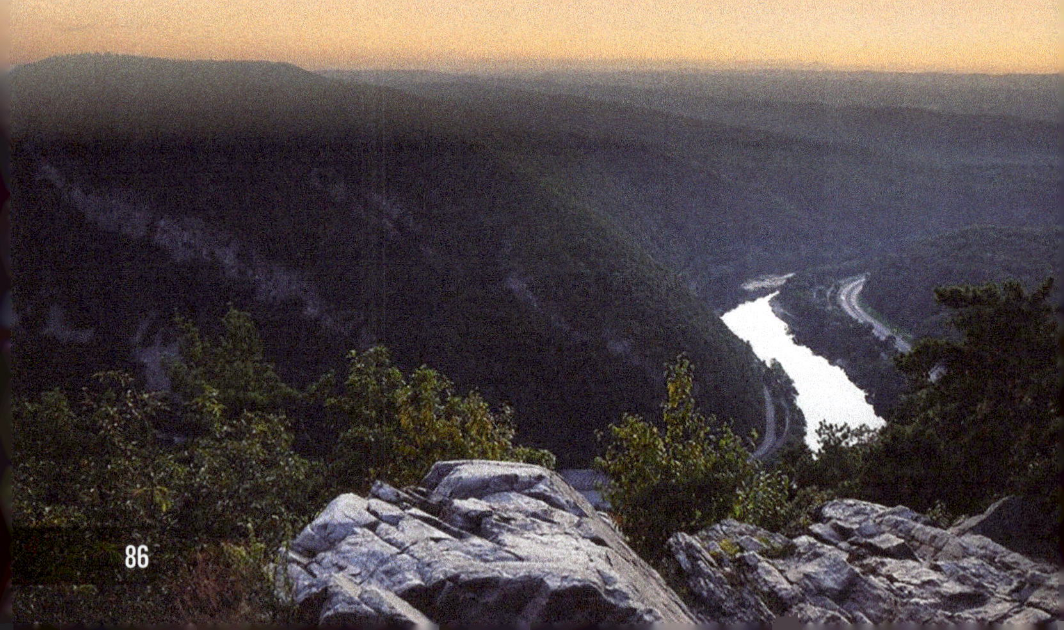

R

Today **I RELEASED** *my... (check all that apply)*

Mind By:
- ■ Communicating my thoughts, feelings, & needs to others
- ■ Speaking positive self-affirmations   ■ Deep breathing   ■ Other _____

Body By:
- ■ Muscle Relaxation Techniques   ■ Exercise
- ■ Hydrotherapy: bath or shower   ■ Other _____

Spirit By:
- ■ Meditation   ■ Journaling   ■ Praying
- ■ Going outside for 15-20 minutes   ■ Self-Talk   ■ Other _____

E

Today **I FEEL**... *(circle one)*

Happy / Anger / Love / Sad / Fear

Surprise / Disgust / Trust / Anticipation

Other _____

What is your dominant **EMOTION** in your life right now?

S

What were your main **STRESSORS** today?

What *Methods* are you using today **TO REDUCE** your current stress?

What *Value* have you noticed **IN USING** them?

T

Stick TOGETHER: How did you *Connect* today?
- ○ Reached out to a co-worker who appeared to be struggling
- ○ Expressed openly with trusted family or co-workers about how the pandemic is affecting me
- ○ Identified factors that are overwhelming/stressful and worked with others to find solutions
- ○ Initiated the "Buddy" System with other co-workers and monitored each other for signs of stress, burnout, and depression
- ○ Spoke to a mental health care provider

My ~~Let's~~ **R.E.S.T.** *Affirmation for Today:*
I rekindle my dreams, gifts, and passions in life. I will accomplish great things.

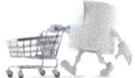 What do you need, but feel like it's unavailable?

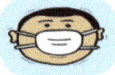 What are you having a hard time expressing?

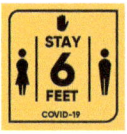 Who or what have you distanced yourself from that could help you overcome the above struggles/difficulties?

 **NEXT STEPS:** Make a healthy plan of action that you will implement in order to help protect yourself from being overtaken by the daily stress of the pandemic. _____
_____
_____
_____
_____
_____
_____

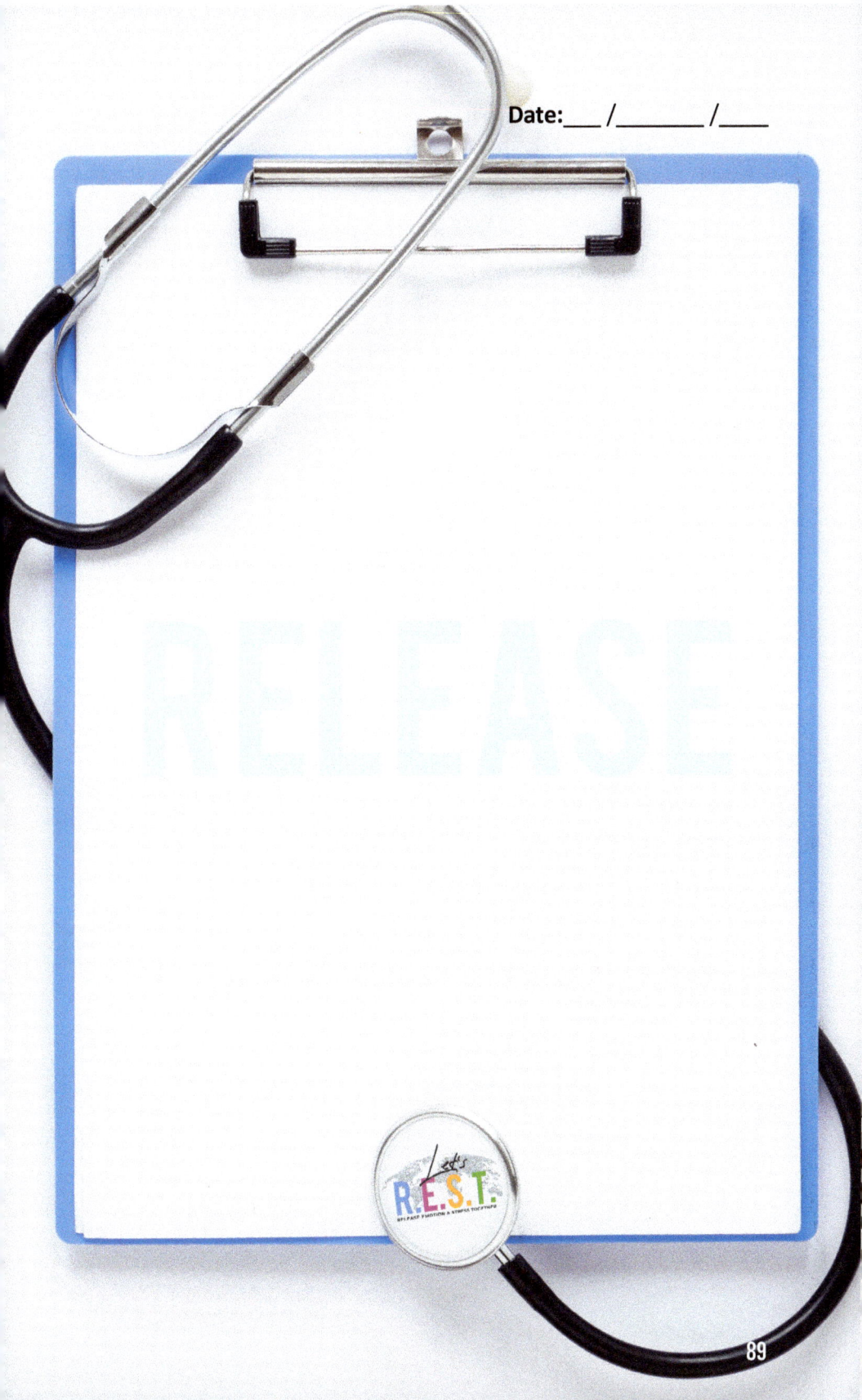

Date:___ / _____ / ___

In order to seize our tomorrow, I believe that we must prepare today.
In preparation for tomorrow, I've discovered
that our todays give many lessons.
When we embrace the lessons of today, we are strengthened
emotionally and physically for our tomorrow.
Therefore, the victory for tomorrow is in the submitting to the
inner change and transformation from the lessons of our today.

--Dr. Chevelta A. Smith

What did you learn **TODAY**, and *how* will you apply this knowledge to become a better/healthier you **TOMORROW?**

Let's R.E.S.T. **Bedtime Affirmation**
(Say it out loud!)

I am strong!
I am resilient!
I am able to overcome every disappointment and setback from today
I am more than a conqueror!
I will recharge myself with good sleep tonight
I will awake with a renewed sense of purpose
And I declare that my tomorrow will be great!

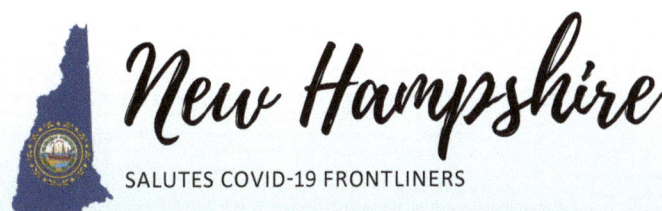

New Hampshire
SALUTES COVID-19 FRONTLINERS

I want to thank all the frontliners out there, who are watching over all our loved ones, and putting their own lives at risk. You are amazing! Thank you for all that you do! We are blessed to have you!

—Lisa W.
Hampton, New Hampshire

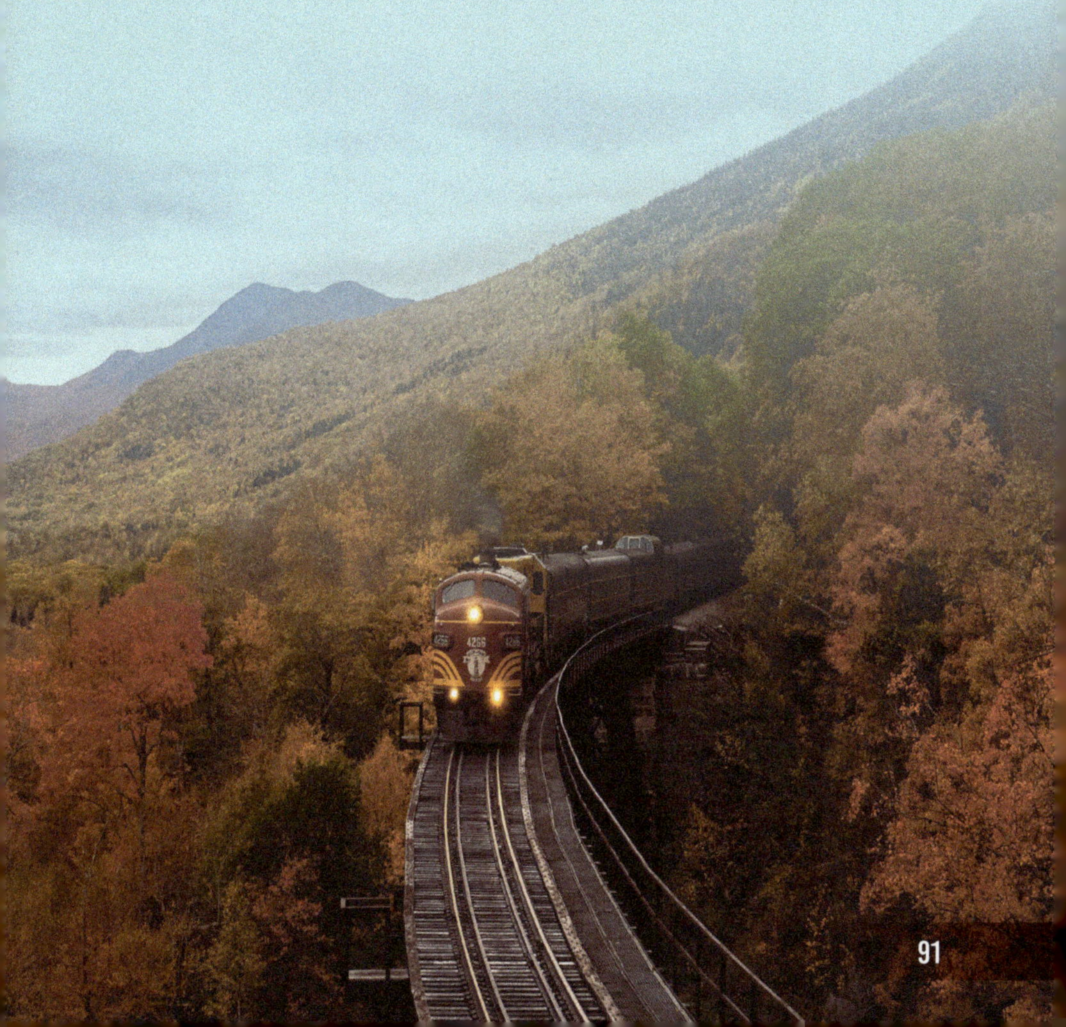

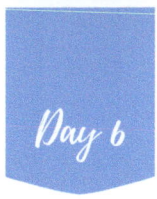

MORNING HUDDLE

When You Serve Others, When You Do Good, When You Give of Yourself—It Will Come Back to You!

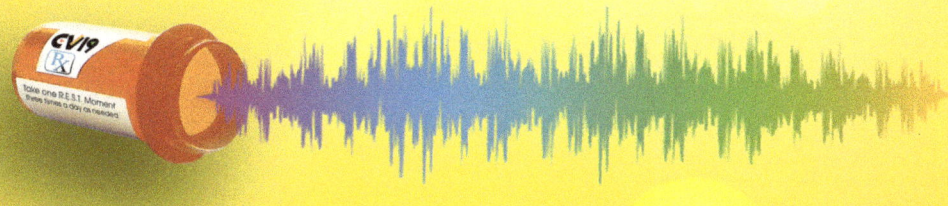

"Give without looking for anything back, knowing that it will come back."

—Dr. Chevelta A. Smith

GIVE

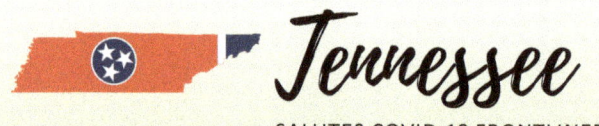

Tennessee
SALUTES COVID-19 FRONTLINERS

In the recent happenings that have shaken the world, the COVID-19 pandemic, we have seen health workers on the frontlines serving selflessly and giving their all to the survival of humanity.
We are encouraged that a reward awaits all of you who continue to do good. We sincerely thank you for sacrificing your time and talent to serve those who were infected with the coronavirus. We appreciate you!

'Let's not become weary in doing good, for at the proper time [you] will reap a harvest if [you] do not give up.'
- Galatians 6:9
We love you! God bless you!

—Dwight & Deidra R.
Nashville, Tennessee

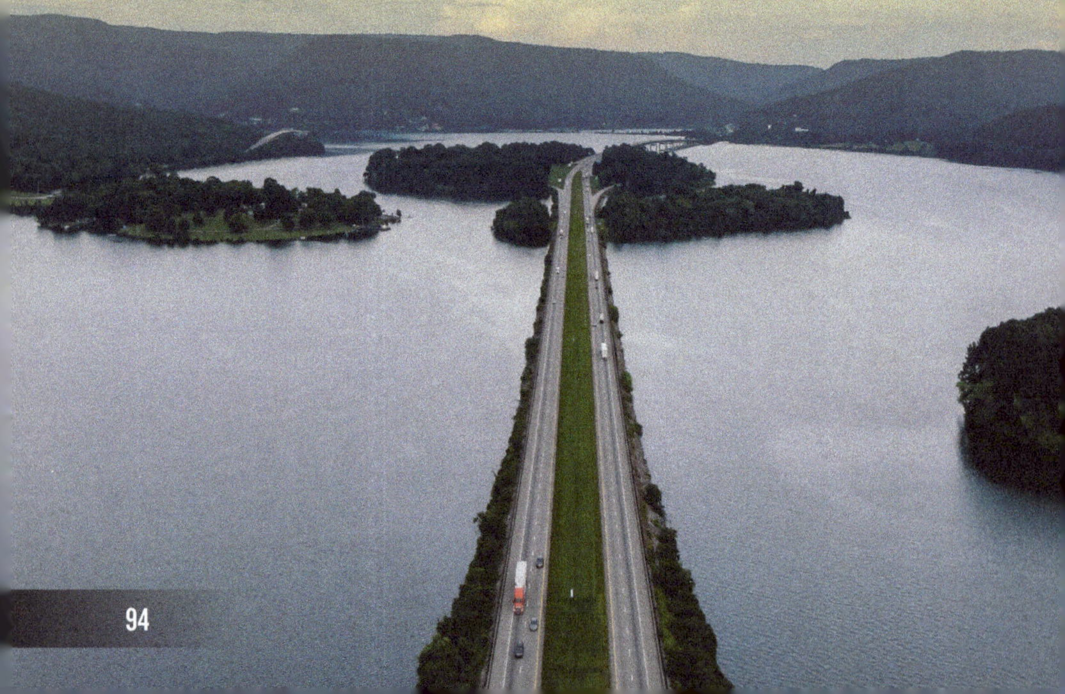

R

Today **I RELEASED** *my... (check all that apply)*

Mind By:
- Communicating my thoughts, feelings, & needs to others
- Speaking positive self-affirmations ■ Deep breathing ■ Other _____

Body By:
- Muscle Relaxation Techniques ■ Exercise
- Hydrotherapy: bath or shower ■ Other _____

Spirit By:
- Meditation ■ Journaling ■ Praying
- Going outside for 15-20 minutes ■ Self-Talk ■ Other _____

E

Today **I FEEL...** *(circle one)*

Happy / Anger / Love / Sad / Fear

Surprise / Disgust / Trust / Anticipation

Other _____

What is your dominant **EMOTION** in your life right now?

S

What were your main **STRESSORS** today?

What *Methods* are you using today **TO REDUCE** your current stress?

What *Value* have you noticed **IN USING** them?

T

Stick TOGETHER: How did you *Connect* today?

- Reached out to a co-worker who appeared to be struggling
- Expressed openly with trusted family or co-workers about how the pandemic is affecting me
- Identified factors that are overwhelming/stressful and worked with others to find solutions
- Initiated the "Buddy" System with other co-workers and monitored each other for signs of stress, burnout, and depression
- Spoke to a mental health care provider

My *Let's* **R.E.S.T.** *Affirmation for Today:*
I have the strength to give selflessly and unconditionally. I am a cheerful giver.

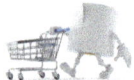
What do you need, but feel like it's unavailable?

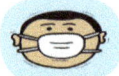
What are you having a hard time expressing?

Who or what have you distanced yourself from that could help you overcome the above struggles/difficulties?

NEXT STEPS: Make a healthy plan of action that you will implement in order to help protect yourself from being overtaken by the daily stress of the pandemic. _____
_____
_____
_____
_____
_____
_____

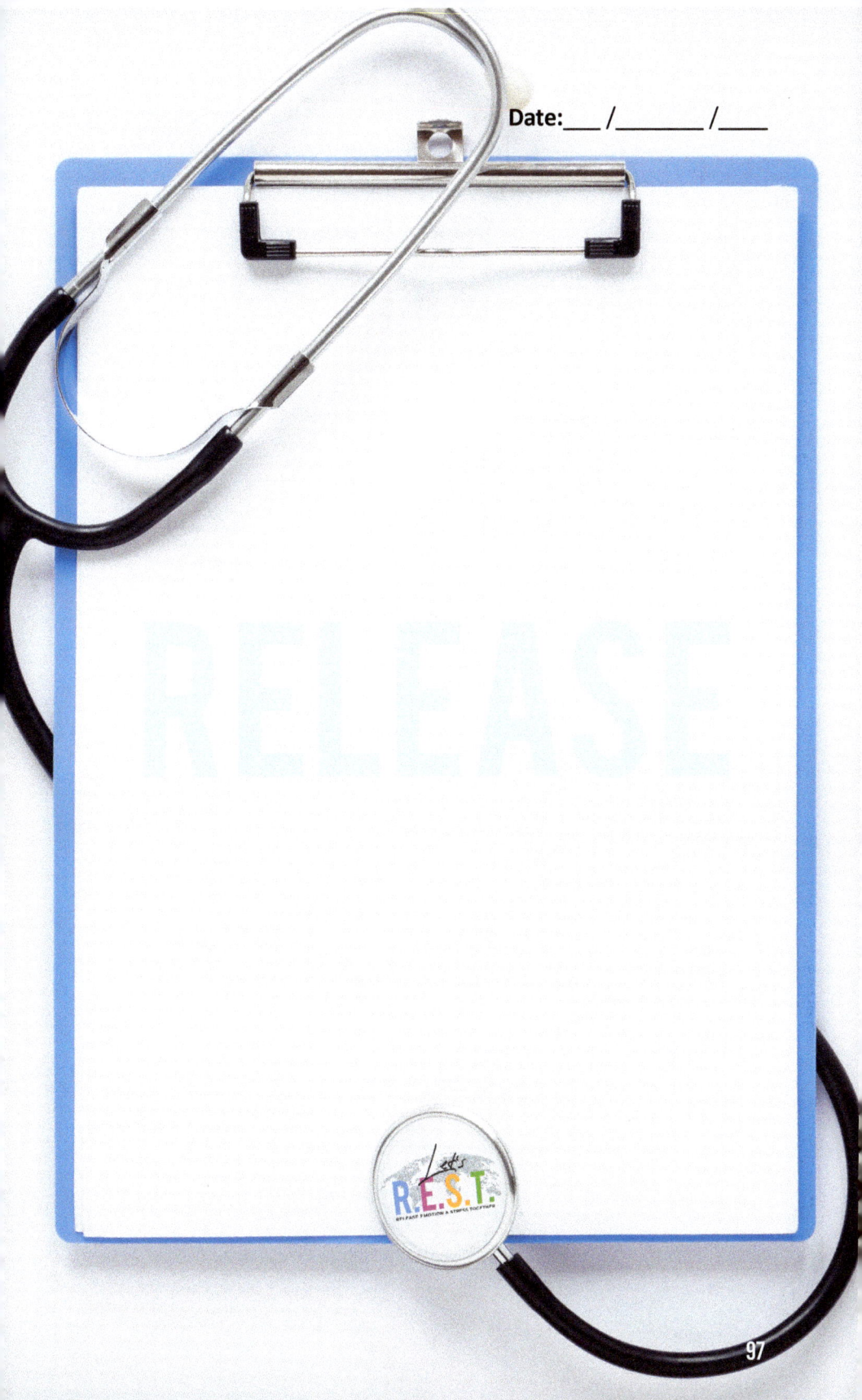
Date:___ / _____ / ___

In order to seize our tomorrow, I believe that we must prepare today.
In preparation for tomorrow, I've discovered
that our todays give many lessons.
When we embrace the lessons of today, we are strengthened
emotionally and physically for our tomorrow.
Therefore, the victory for tomorrow is in the submitting to the
inner change and transformation from the lessons of our today.

--Dr. Chevelta A. Smith

What did you learn **TODAY,** and *how* will you apply this knowledge to become a better/healthier you **TOMORROW?**

Let's R.E.S.T. **Bedtime Affirmation**
(Say it out loud!)

I am strong!
I am resilient!
I am able to overcome every disappointment and setback from today
I am more than a conqueror!
I will recharge myself with good sleep tonight
I will awake with a renewed sense of purpose
And I declare that my tomorrow will be great!

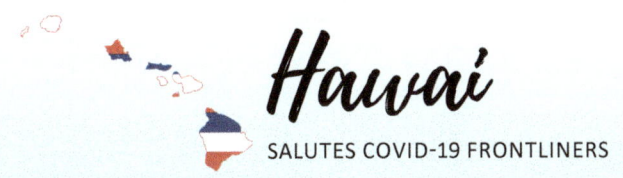

Hawai'i
SALUTES COVID-19 FRONTLINERS

I cannot begin to explain how grateful I am for every single first responder and essential worker. Thank you for being selfless; thank you for caring for others above yourself; thank you for not giving up; thank you for staying patient with all of us; thank you for putting in the long hours; thank you for showing up consistently; and thank you for just being there. We would be lost without your selflessness. We owe everything to you all. Thank you will never be enough.
With so much love, I thank you from Hawaii!

—*Renee B.*
Hawaii

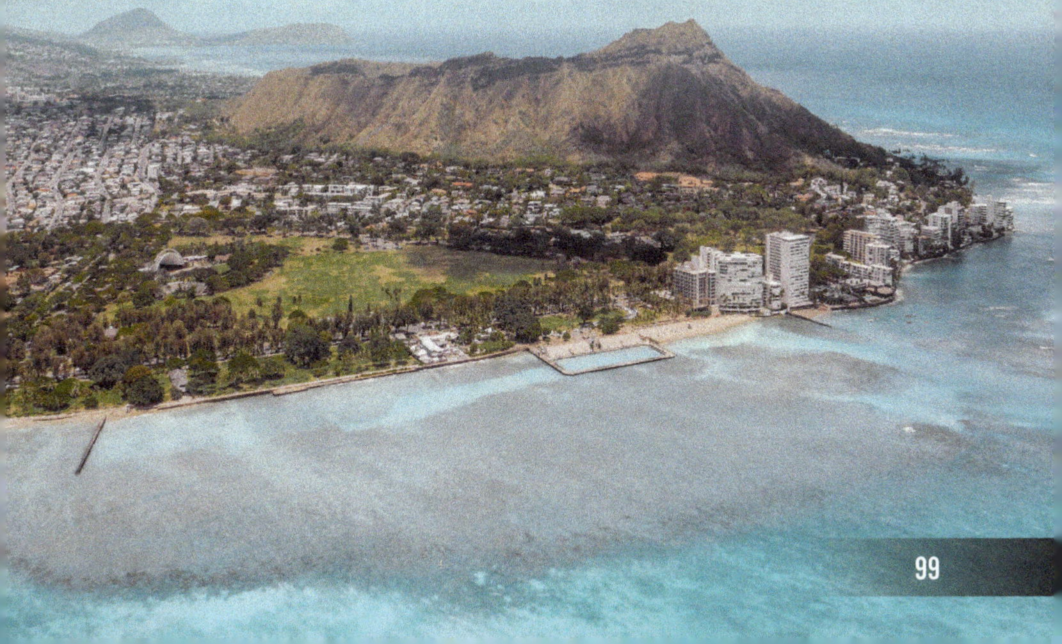

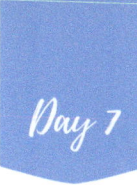

Day 7

MORNING HUDDLE

You Must Be Intentional About Everything You Do in Your Day. Do Everything With an Intention to Be Successful.

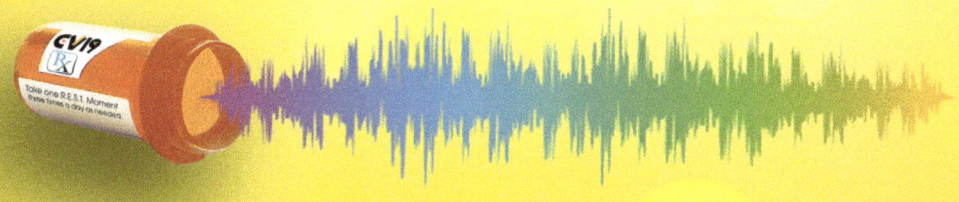

"Attack your day intentionally, not haphazardly."
—Dr. Chevelta A. Smith

INTENTIONAL

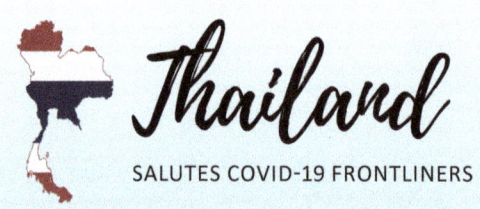

Thailand
SALUTES COVID-19 FRONTLINERS

我想感谢世界所的医护人员和卫生保健工作者。我希望所有医护人员在照顾病人的同时，也能保护好自己，因为在这个疫情之中，奔在最前线的是你们。你们真的是世界的英雄！感谢他们的辛劳，希望这次疫情赶快结束。

—Alice
Bangkok, Thailand

(English Translation):
Thank you to all the incredible, brave medical frontliners of this COVID-19 pandemic. You've done so much in this crisis and sacrificed even more, and for that, this world can't thank you enough. I hope that you and your families all remain safe, and I'll keep you all in my prayers. Thank you.

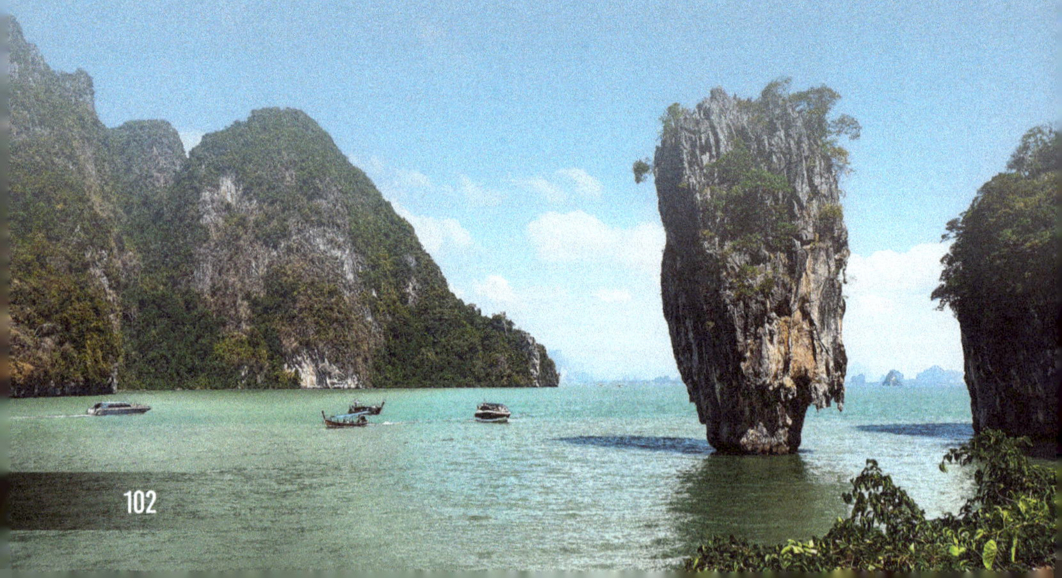

R

Today I RELEASED my... (check all that apply)

Mind By:
- Communicating my thoughts, feelings, & needs to others
- Speaking positive self-affirmations
- Deep breathing
- Other _____

Body By:
- Muscle Relaxation Techniques
- Exercise
- Hydrotherapy: bath or shower
- Other _____

Spirit By:
- Meditation
- Journaling
- Praying
- Going outside for 15-20 minutes
- Self-Talk
- Other _____

E

Today I FEEL... (circle one)

Happy / Anger / Love / Sad / Fear

Surprise / Disgust / Trust / Anticipation

Other_____

What is your dominant **EMOTION** in your life right now?

S

What were your main **STRESSORS** today?

What *Methods* are you using today **TO REDUCE** your current stress?

What *Value* have you noticed **IN USING** them?

T

Stick TOGETHER: How did you *Connect* today?

- Reached out to a co-worker who appeared to be struggling
- Expressed openly with trusted family or co-workers about how the pandemic is affecting me
- Identified factors that are overwhelming/stressful and worked with others to find solutions
- Initiated the "Buddy" System with other co-workers and monitored each other for signs of stress, burnout, and depression
- Spoke to a mental health care provider

My *Let's* R.E.S.T. *Affirmation for Today:*

I will be intentional in my life and live wisely. I will make the most of my time and use it to fulfill my purpose.

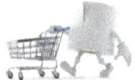 What do you need, but feel like it's unavailable?

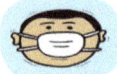 What are you having a hard time expressing?

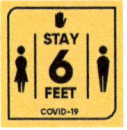 Who or what have you distanced yourself from that could help you overcome the above struggles/difficulties?

 **NEXT STEPS:** Make a healthy plan of action that you will implement in order to help protect yourself from being overtaken by the daily stress of the pandemic. _____
_____
_____
_____
_____
_____
_____

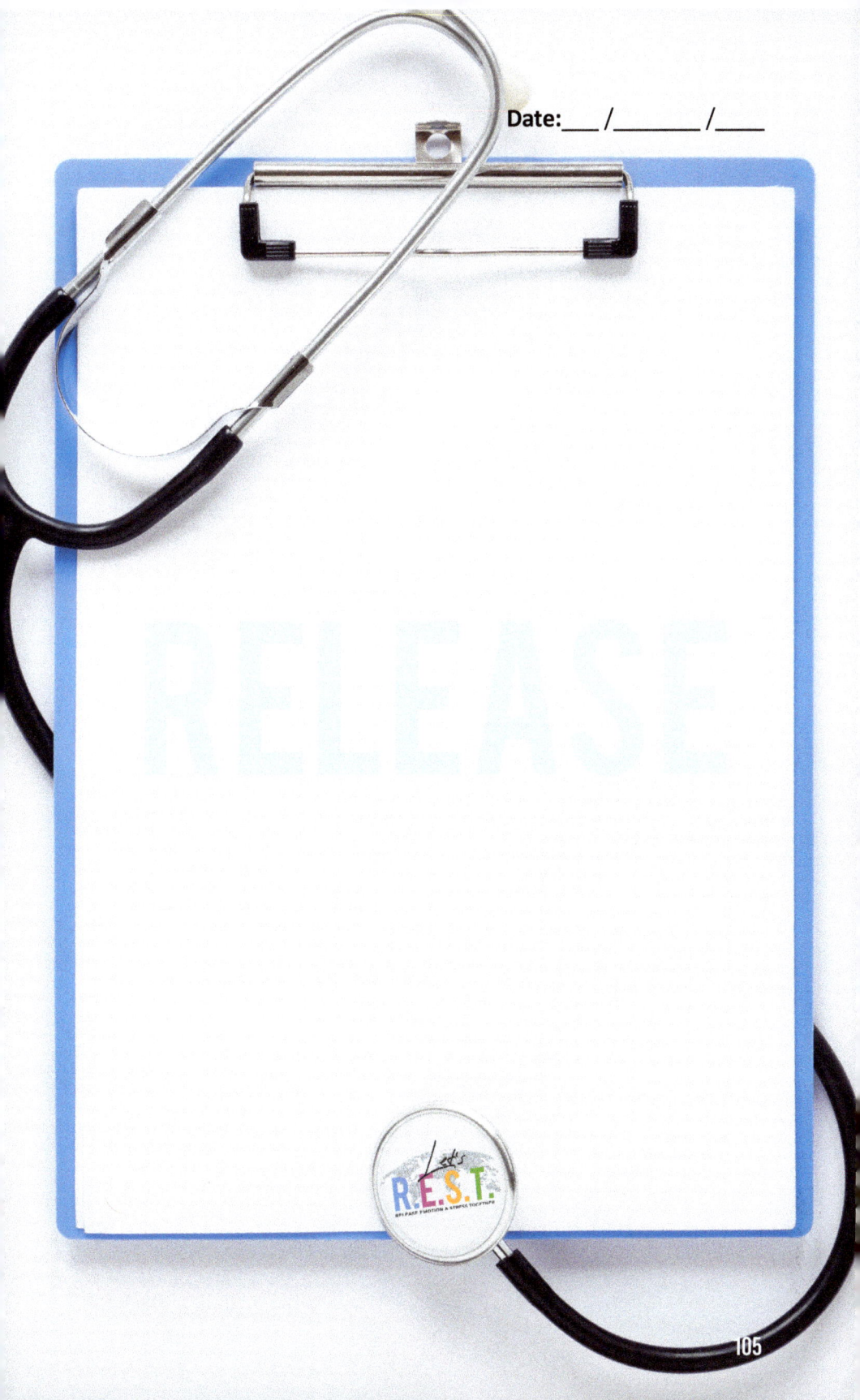

In order to seize our tomorrow, I believe that we must prepare today.
In preparation for tomorrow, I've discovered
that our todays give many lessons.
When we embrace the lessons of today, we are strengthened
emotionally and physically for our tomorrow.
Therefore, the victory for tomorrow is in the submitting to the
inner change and transformation from the lessons of our today.

‑‑Dr. Chevelta A. Smith

What did you learn **TODAY**, and *how* will you apply this knowledge to become a better/healthier you **TOMORROW?**

Let's R.E.S.T. **Bedtime Affirmation**
(Say it out loud!)

I am strong!
I am resilient!
I am able to overcome every disappointment and setback from today
I am more than a conqueror!
I will recharge myself with good sleep tonight
I will awake with a renewed sense of purpose
And I declare that my tomorrow will be great!

US Virgin Islands

SALUTES COVID-19 FRONTLINERS

Sam, the sailor, was refused entry by many ports but, The Honorable Governor, Albert Bryan, accepted him into the US Virgin Islands because it was the right thing to do. Twelve weeks later, he has recovered from COVID-19. This is the essence of who we are as a Virgin Islands people.

During this season of COVID-19, it is comforting to know those frontline workers (doctors, nurses, LPN's, CNA's, security staff, kitchen staff, office workers) are dedicated to their professions and serve with excellence. Thank you.

—Leonilda BJ
St Thomas, US Virgin Islands

I can do all things through Christ who strengthens me!

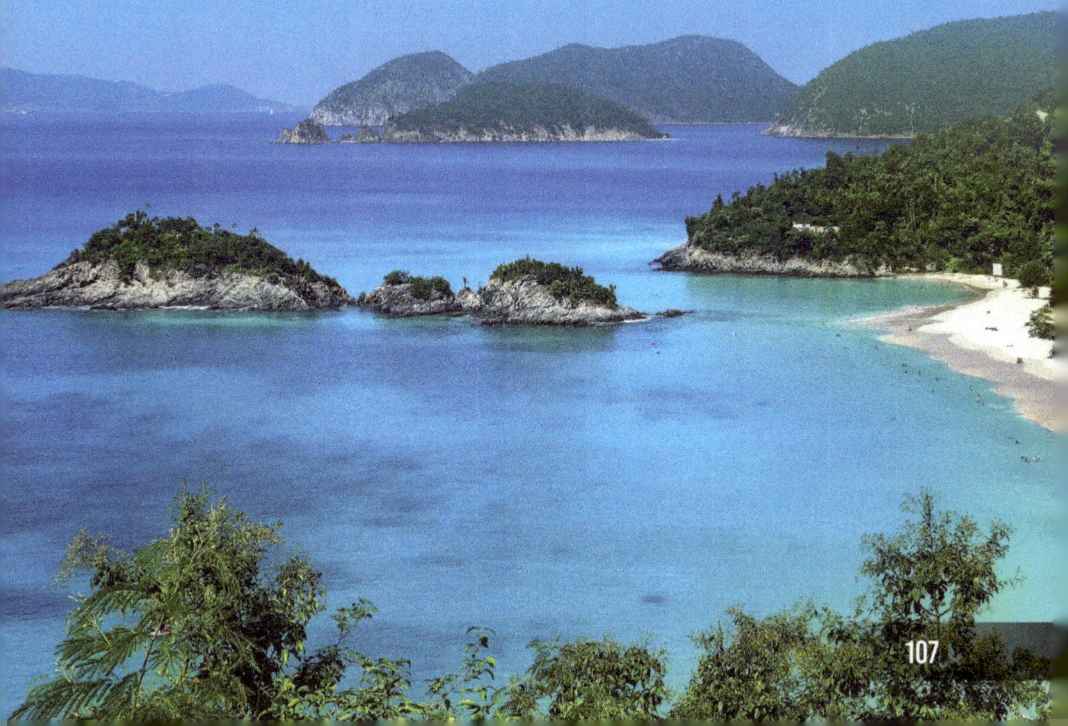

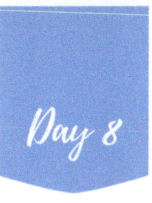

Day 8

MORNING HUDDLE

Accept That You Are Great. Believe That You Are Great. Then, Begin to Walk in the Confidence of Your Greatness.

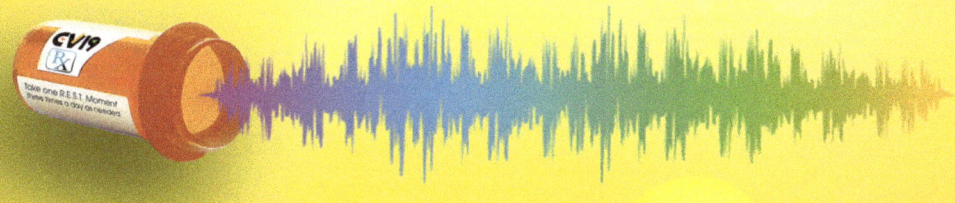

"You don't have to make an apology for being great!"
—Dr. Chevelta A. Smith

AFFIRMATION CONFIDENCE

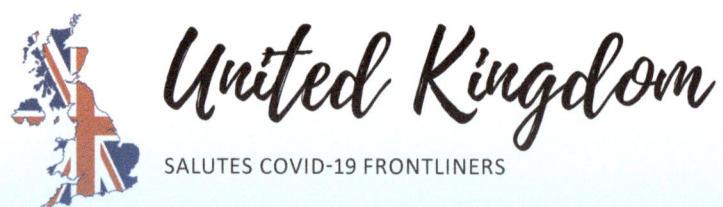

United Kingdom

SALUTES COVID-19 FRONTLINERS

Front and line are two words that (in and of themselves) say so much. In battle, a frontliner is considered the bravest and most admired. He acts as a shield for those who are behind him.

You have done just that and for that, we are forever grateful. I have a prayer for you, Dear Frontliner; that everything that you had to risk and give up, that God will restore to you 100 fold and that although you had to put on your brave face, my prayer is that you will always know God to be your brave and safe place.

Love you Frontliner,

*—Tobi A.
London, England
United Kingdom*

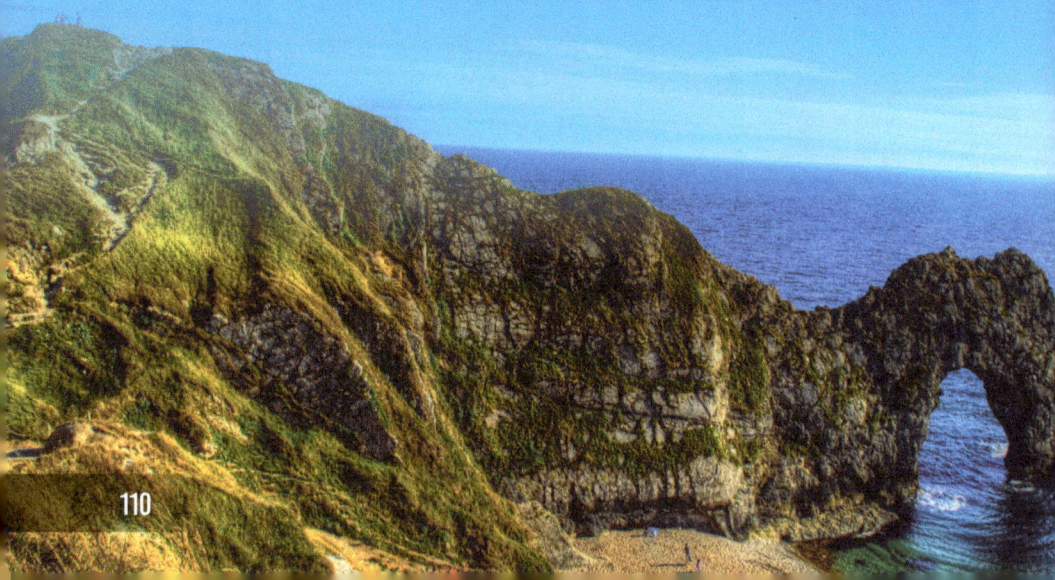

R

Today I RELEASED my... (check all that apply)

Mind By:
- Communicating my thoughts, feelings, & needs to others
- Speaking positive self-affirmations
- Deep breathing
- Other _____

Body By:
- Muscle Relaxation Techniques
- Exercise
- Hydrotherapy: bath or shower
- Other _____

Spirit By:
- Meditation
- Journaling
- Praying
- Going outside for 15-20 minutes
- Self-Talk
- Other _____

E

Today I FEEL... (circle one)

Happy / Anger / Love / Sad / Fear

Surprise / Disgust / Trust / Anticipation

Other_____

What is your dominant EMOTION in your life right now?

S

What were your main STRESSORS today?

What *Methods* are you using today TO REDUCE your current stress?

What *Value* have you noticed IN USING them?

T

Stick TOGETHER: How did you *Connect* today?

- Reached out to a co-worker who appeared to be struggling
- Expressed openly with trusted family or co-workers about how the pandemic is affecting me
- Identified factors that are overwhelming/stressful and worked with others to find solutions
- Initiated the "Buddy" System with other co-workers and monitored each other for signs of stress, burnout, and depression
- Spoke to a mental health care provider

My *Let's* R.E.S.T. Affirmation for Today:
I have everything in me that I need to be successful! I am confident that I will not fail!

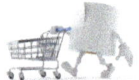 What do you need, but feel like it's unavailable?

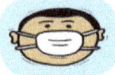 What are you having a hard time expressing?

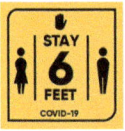 Who or what have you distanced yourself from that could help you overcome the above struggles/difficulties?

 **NEXT STEPS:** Make a healthy plan of action that you will implement in order to help protect yourself from being overtaken by the daily stress of the pandemic. _____
_____
_____
_____
_____
_____
_____

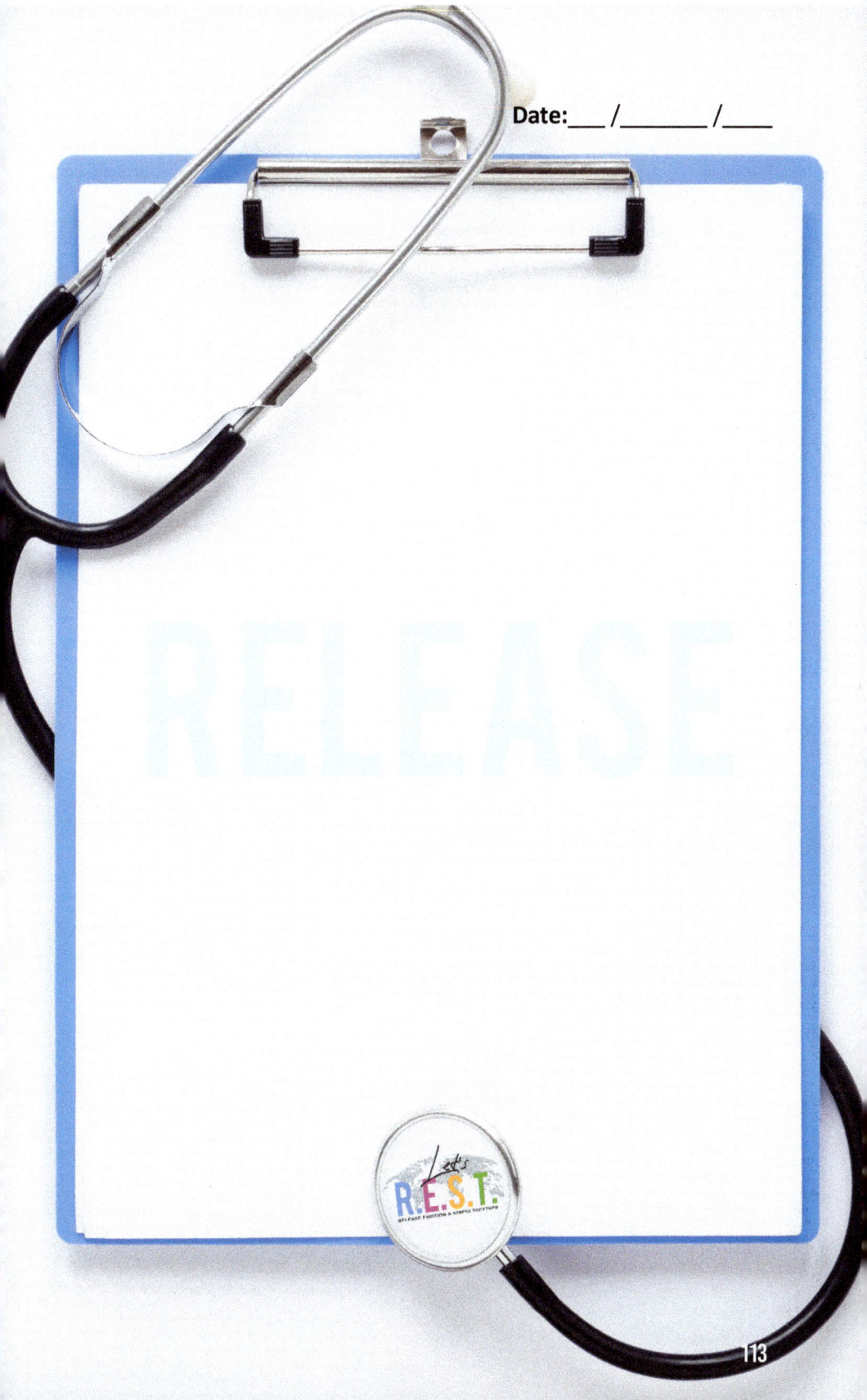

In order to seize our tomorrow, I believe that we must prepare today.
In preparation for tomorrow, I've discovered
that our todays give many lessons.
When we embrace the lessons of today, we are strengthened
emotionally and physically for our tomorrow.
Therefore, the victory for tomorrow is in the submitting to the
inner change and transformation from the lessons of our today.

--Dr. Chevelta A. Smith

What did you learn **TODAY**, and *how* will you apply this knowledge to become a better/healthier you **TOMORROW?**

Let's R.E.S.T. **Bedtime Affirmation**
(Say it out loud!)

I am strong!
I am resilient!
I am able to overcome every disappointment and setback from today
I am more than a conqueror!
I will recharge myself with good sleep tonight
I will awake with a renewed sense of purpose
And I declare that my tomorrow will be great!

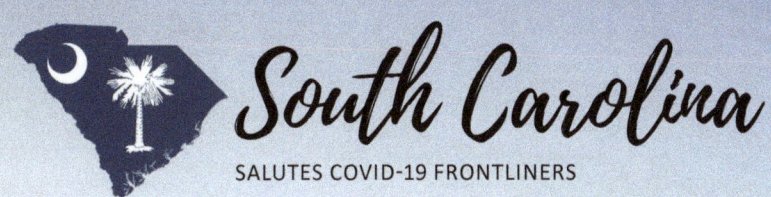

South Carolina
SALUTES COVID-19 FRONTLINERS

No one can fully comprehend what it takes to get up every morning with the knowledge that the tasks ahead are practically unbearable. The concern for your patients, your family, and yourself is ever-present, yet you press through exhaustion and concerns each day to save lives. We will never be able to thank you for this - for the many sacrifices. And with tears in our eyes and gratitude in our hearts, we ask God to cover you, to build you up on every side, and to provide miracles for you and those in your care.

—Dorothy J.
Summerville, South Carolina

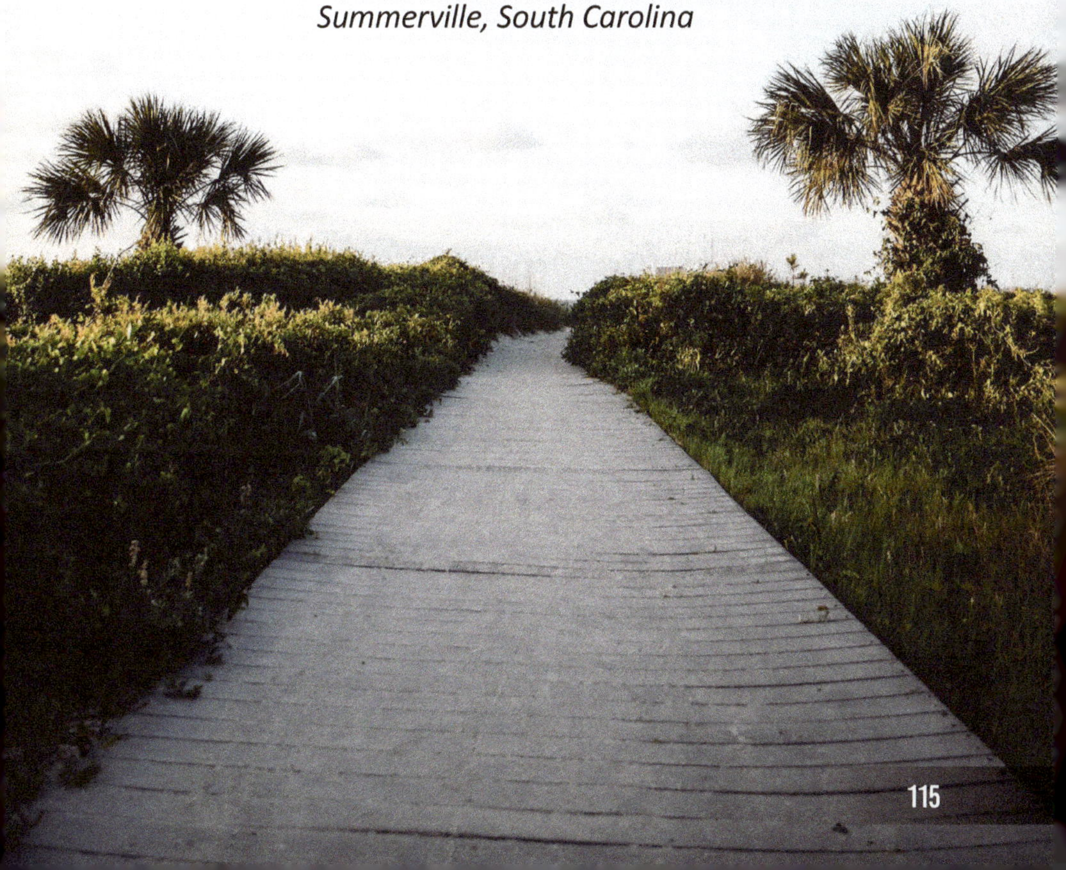

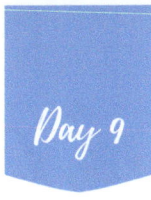

Day 9

MORNING HUDDLE

We Are Not Supermans Flying Around With Capes. We Are Not Batmans in the Batmobile. We Are Human Beings, and as Human Beings, We All Have Areas in Which We Will Need the Assistance of Others.

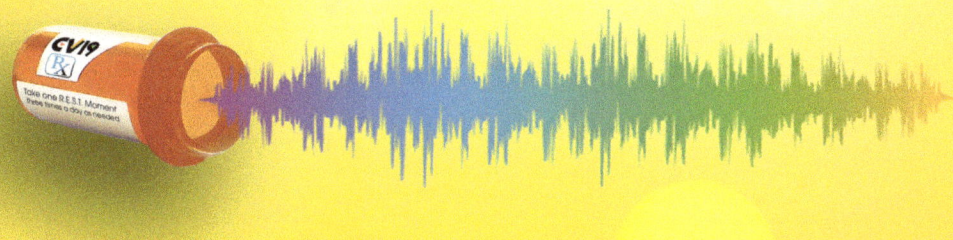

"You've got the umph inside of you to overcome every obstacle."

—Dr. Chevelta A. Smith

STEADFAST

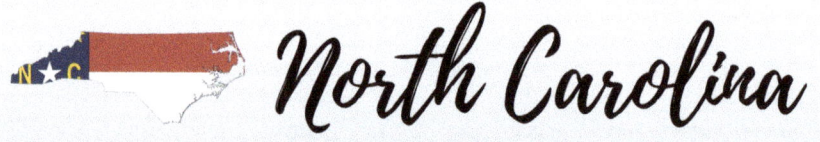
North Carolina
SALUTES COVID-19 FRONTLINERS

...And let the peace of God guard your heart & mind through Christ Jesus! Be ye steadfast, unmovable, Always abounding in the work of the Lord, knowing your labor is not in vain! I pray for you frontline workers always! Go with God & may God go before you!

—Sidney & Cathy O.
Charlotte, North Carolina

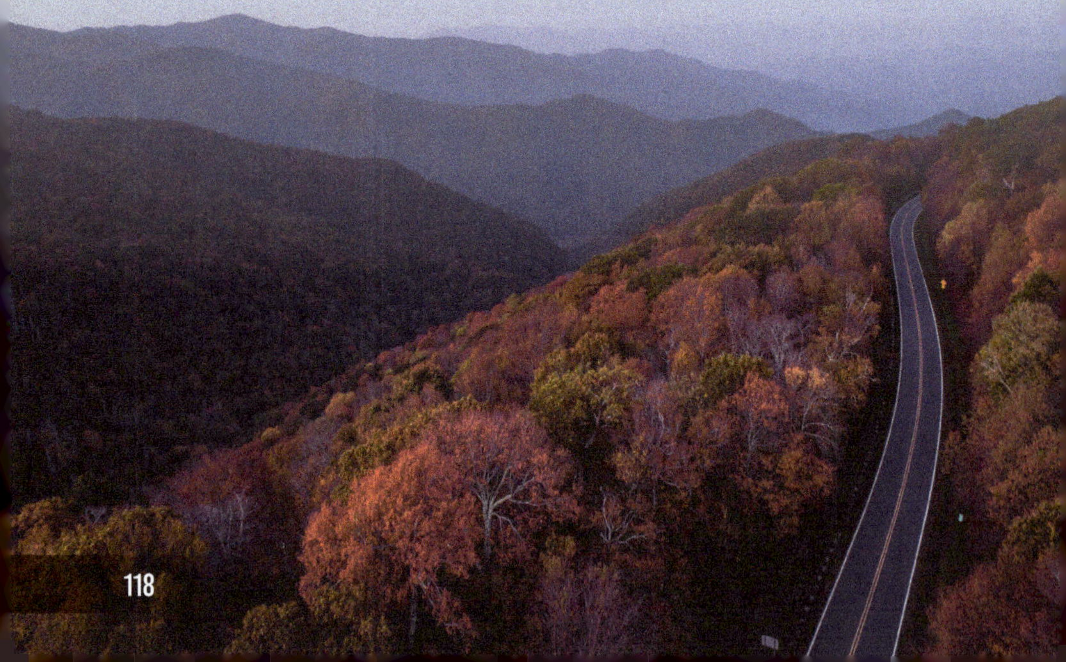

R — Today **I RELEASED** *my*... (check all that apply)

Mind By:
- ☐ Communicating my thoughts, feelings, & needs to others
- ☐ Speaking positive self-affirmations ☐ Deep breathing ☐ Other _____

Body By:
- ☐ Muscle Relaxation Techniques   ☐ Exercise
- ☐ Hydrotherapy: bath or shower   ☐ Other _____

Spirit By:
- ☐ Meditation   ☐ Journaling   ☐ Praying
- ☐ Going outside for 15-20 minutes   ☐ Self-Talk   ☐ Other _____

E — Today **I FEEL**... *(circle one)*

Happy / Anger / Love / Sad / Fear

Surprise / Disgust / Trust / Anticipation

Other _____

What is your dominant **EMOTION** in your life right now?

S

What were your main **STRESSORS** today?

What *Methods* are you using today **TO REDUCE** your current stress?

What *Value* have you noticed **IN USING** them?

T — Stick **TOGETHER**: How did you *Connect* today?

- ○ Reached out to a co-worker who appeared to be struggling
- ○ Expressed openly with trusted family or co-workers about how the pandemic is affecting me
- ○ Identified factors that are overwhelming/stressful and worked with others to find solutions
- ○ Initiated the "Buddy" System with other co-workers and monitored each other for signs of stress, burnout, and depression
- ○ Spoke to a mental health care provider

My *Let's* **R.E.S.T.** *Affirmation for Today:*
I am full of grit! I will be steadfast and strong in every challenge I face today.

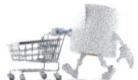 What do you need, but feel like it's unavailable?

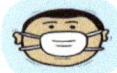 What are you having a hard time expressing?

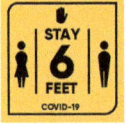 Who or what have you distanced yourself from that could help you overcome the above struggles/difficulties?

 **NEXT STEPS: Make a healthy plan of action that you will implement in order to help protect yourself from being overtaken by the daily stress of the pandemic.** _____
_____
_____
_____
_____
_____
_____

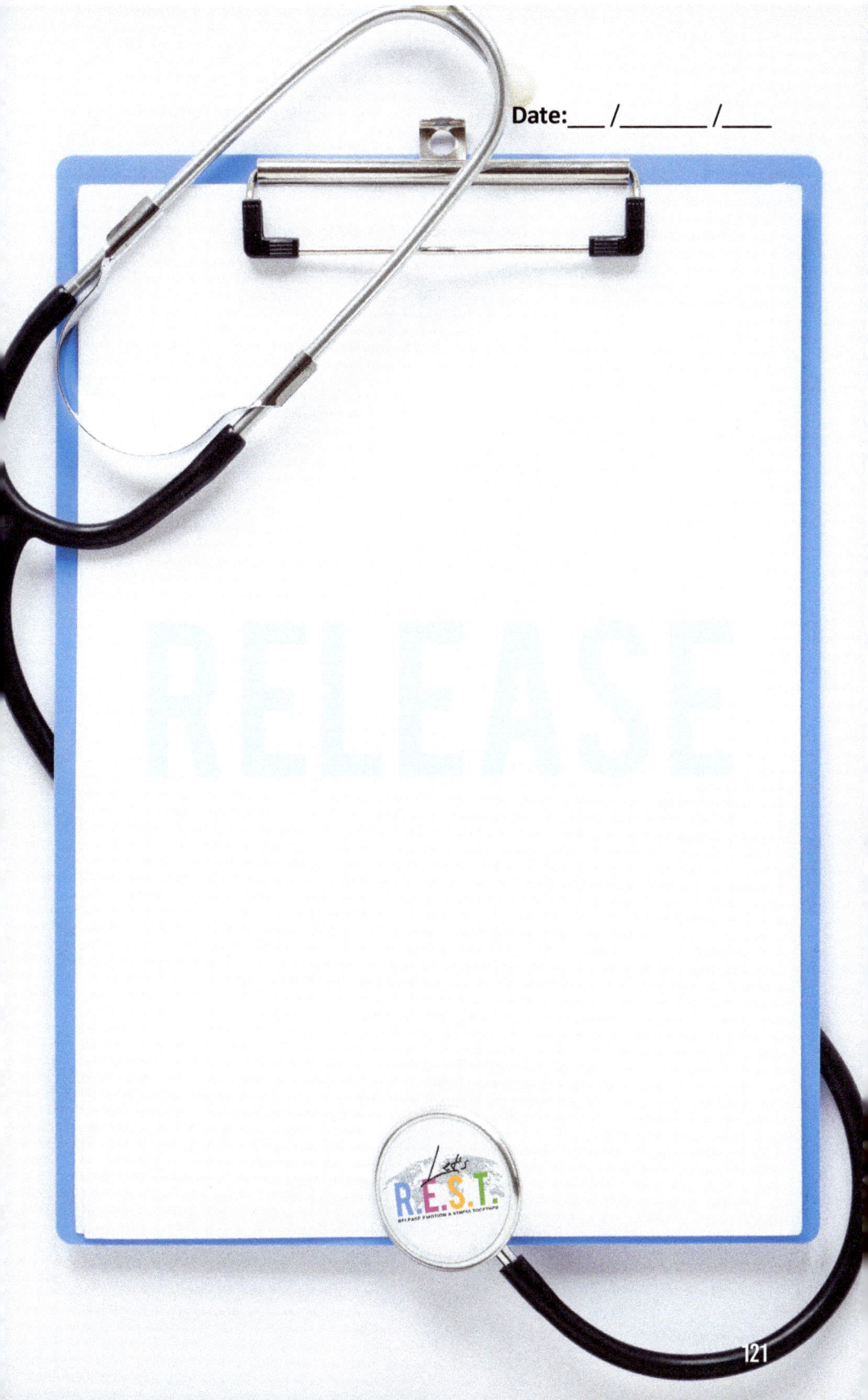

In order to seize our tomorrow, I believe that we must prepare today.
In preparation for tomorrow, I've discovered
that our todays give many lessons.
When we embrace the lessons of today, we are strengthened
emotionally and physically for our tomorrow.
Therefore, the victory for tomorrow is in the submitting to the
inner change and transformation from the lessons of our today.

--Dr. Chevelta A. Smith

What did you learn **TODAY**, and *how* will you apply this knowledge to become a better/healthier you **TOMORROW?**

Let's R.E.S.T. **Bedtime Affirmation**
(Say it out loud!)

I am strong!
I am resilient!
I am able to overcome every disappointment and setback from today
I am more than a conqueror!
I will recharge myself with good sleep tonight
I will awake with a renewed sense of purpose
And I declare that my tomorrow will be great!

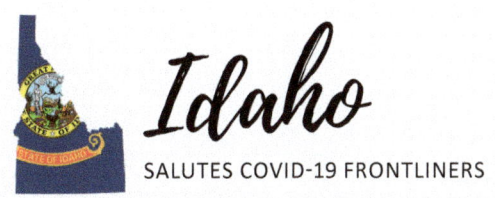

Idaho
SALUTES COVID-19 FRONTLINERS

Frontline healthcare workers are like educators in that we each have a calling. We work tirelessly to meet the needs of the world's most vulnerable population. For educators, it is our students but for you, it is the ever-increasing number of patients who are inflicted with a virus for which, there is no known prevention, nor cure.

Thank you for placing other's needs before your own and for truly making a difference for so many. You are not alone and you are appreciated more than you will ever know.

—Anonymous
Meridian, Idaho

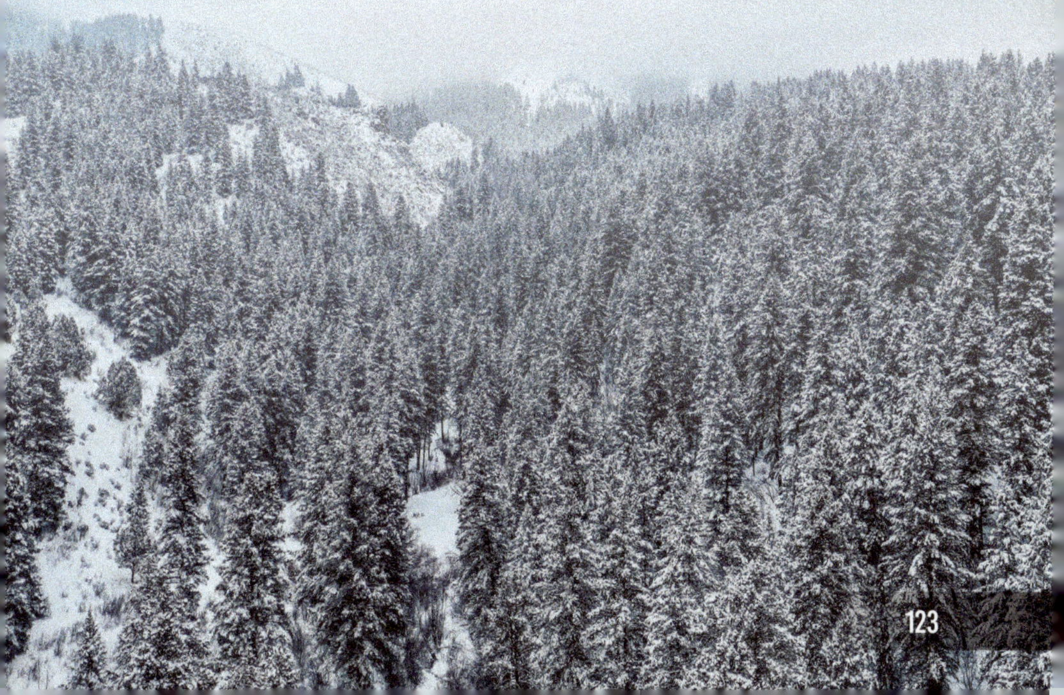

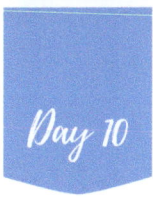

Day 10

MORNING HUDDLE

What God Has Placed in Us to Birth to This World (Gifts, Talents, and Dreams) Is Often Big. As a Result, He Will Intentionally Place Others in Our Lives to Help Us Initiate the Process of Delivering It.

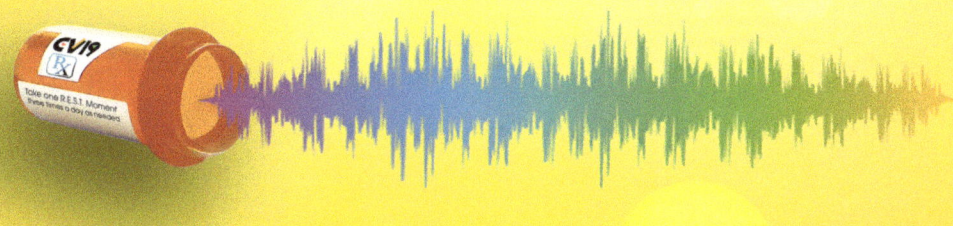

"What God has placed in you to birth is bigger than you. As a result, you need a team to help you bring it forth."

—Dr. Chevelta A. Smith

INDUCE

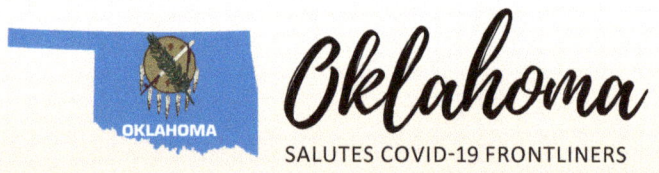

Oklahoma
SALUTES COVID-19 FRONTLINERS

To the Frontliners of COVID-19...
Words cannot express my gratitude. As a daughter of a current OB/Gyn frontliner, I salute you. I have watched my beautiful mother risk her life while delivering children of COVID-19 infected mothers during this pandemic. Despite the loss this virus has caused, she is a constant reminder that life continues. So remember that yes, the loss can be overwhelming during this time, but hold tight to the birthing that's happening in the midst of it all.

—Brookelynn S.
Tulsa, Oklahoma

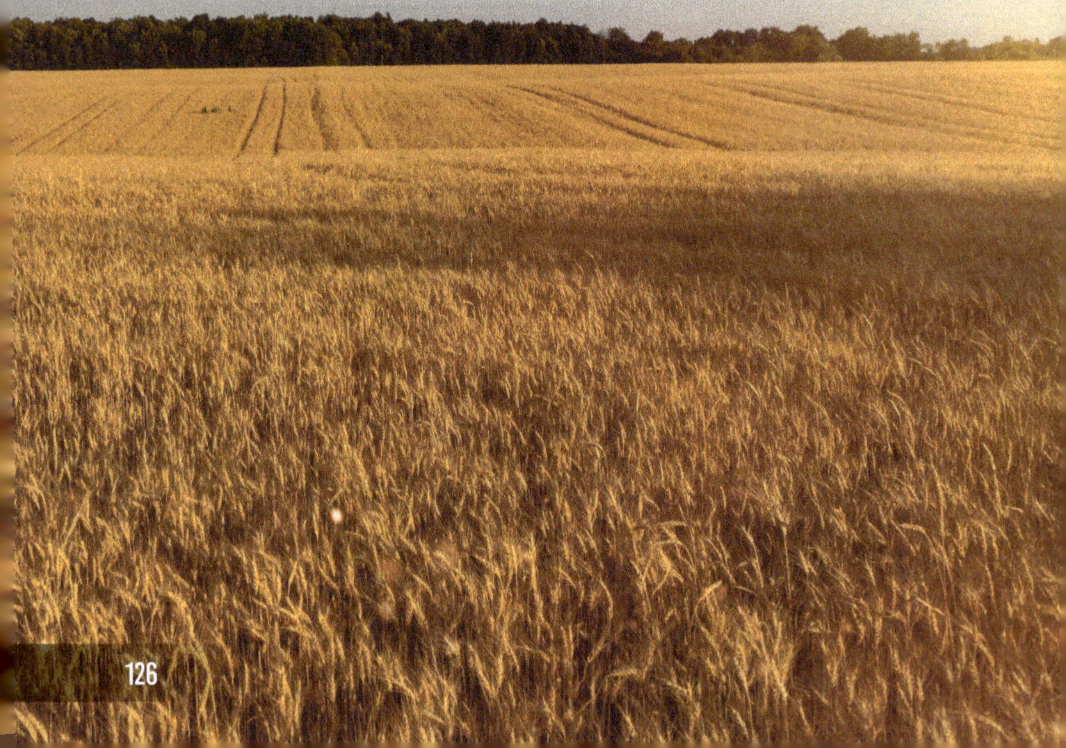

R — Today **I RELEASED** my... *(check all that apply)*

Mind By:
- Communicating my thoughts, feelings, & needs to others
- Speaking positive self-affirmations
- Deep breathing
- Other _____

Body By:
- Muscle Relaxation Techniques
- Exercise
- Hydrotherapy: bath or shower
- Other _____

Spirit By:
- Meditation
- Journaling
- Praying
- Going outside for 15-20 minutes
- Self-Talk
- Other _____

E — Today **I FEEL**... *(circle one)*

Happy / Anger / Love / Sad / Fear

Surprise / Disgust / Trust / Anticipation

Other _____

What is your dominant **EMOTION** in your life right now?

S

What were your main **STRESSORS** today?

What *Methods* are you using today **TO REDUCE** your current stress?

What *Value* have you noticed **IN USING** them?

T — Stick **TOGETHER**: How did you *Connect* today?

- Reached out to a co-worker who appeared to be struggling
- Expressed openly with trusted family or co-workers about how the pandemic is affecting me
- Identified factors that are overwhelming/stressful and worked with others to find solutions
- Initiated the "Buddy" System with other co-workers and monitored each other for signs of stress, burnout, and depression
- Spoke to a mental health care provider

My *Let's* **R.E.S.T.** *Affirmation for Today:*

I have greatness inside of me that is a blessing to others. I am full of life. I have the capacity to produce joy.

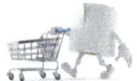 What do you need, but feel like it's unavailable?

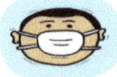 What are you having a hard time expressing?

 Who or what have you distanced yourself from that could help you overcome the above struggles/difficulties?

 NEXT STEPS: Make a healthy plan of action that you will implement in order to help protect yourself from being overtaken by the daily stress of the pandemic. _____
_____
_____
_____
_____
_____
_____

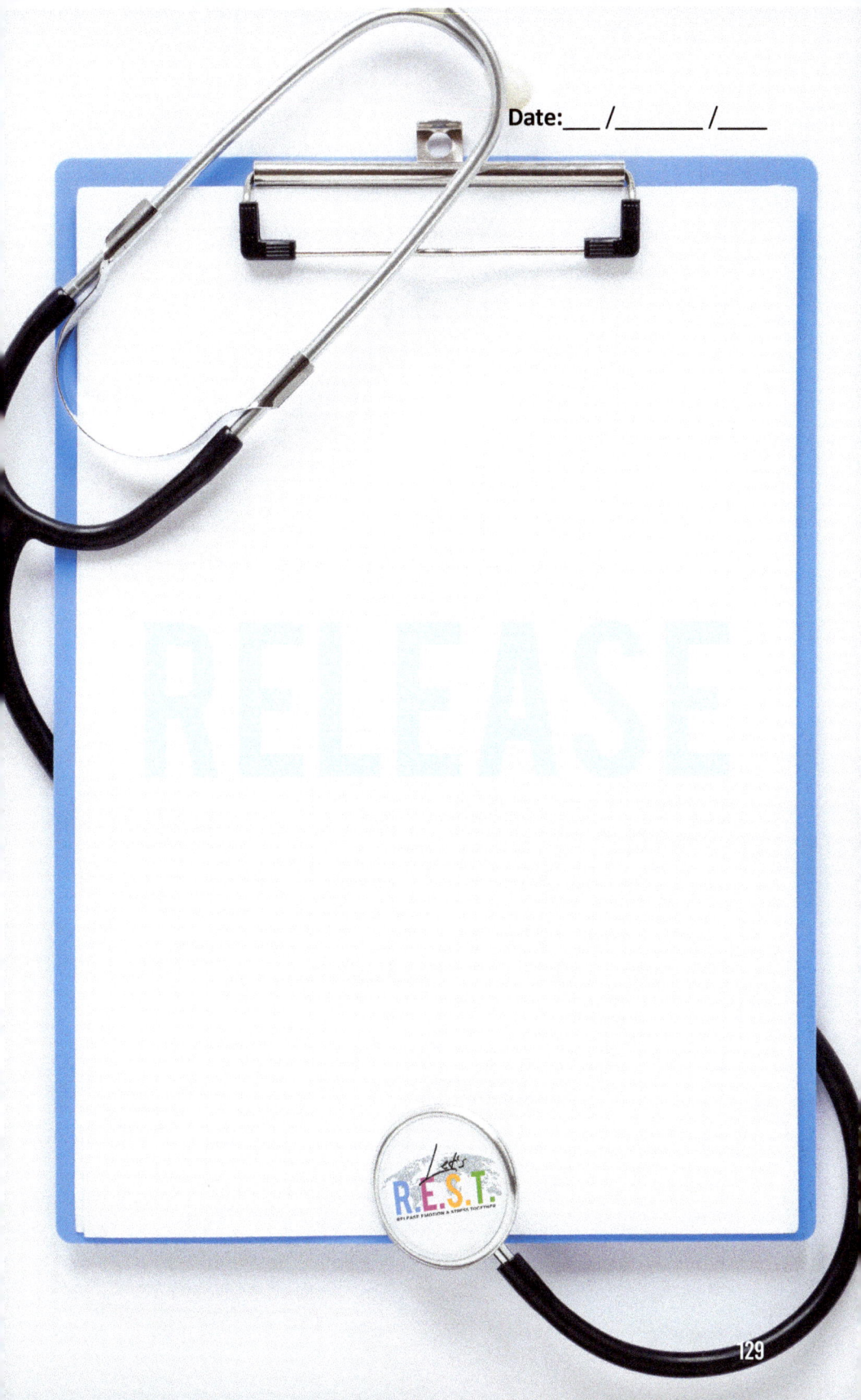

In order to seize our tomorrow, I believe that we must prepare today.
In preparation for tomorrow, I've discovered
that our todays give many lessons.
When we embrace the lessons of today, we are strengthened
emotionally and physically for our tomorrow.
Therefore, the victory for tomorrow is in the submitting to the
inner change and transformation from the lessons of our today.

— —Dr. Chevelta A. Smith

What did you learn **TODAY,** and *how* will you apply this knowledge to become a better/healthier you **TOMORROW?**

Let's R.E.S.T. **Bedtime Affirmation**
(Say it out loud!)

I am strong!
I am resilient!
I am able to overcome every disappointment and setback from today
I am more than a conqueror!
I will recharge myself with good sleep tonight
I will awake with a renewed sense of purpose
And I declare that my tomorrow will be great!

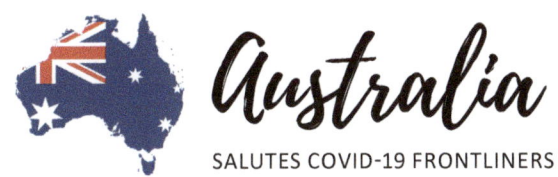

Australia
SALUTES COVID-19 FRONTLINERS

Who would have ever imagined that this beautiful world we live in is at war with an invisible enemy? Who would have ever imagined that our lives are solely in the hands of one unique group of people?

These people do not carry guns and will never fire a bullet. These people are only armed with knowledge, determination, resilience, inner strength, and complete respect for human life. This group of people suffer devastating setbacks, but they will never give up the fight. Unlike other past wars, no medals will be handed out at the end of this battle to the heroes who fought to save lives... our lives.

Therefore, we give our thanks, respect, love, and encouragement to this incredible group of people. They are fighting a battle with every part of their being, not with man-made weapons. It is the hearts, minds, and souls of our first responders and frontline healthcare workers who have fought this invisible enemy and continue to do so. You are truly inspirational. Our world would be a very different place without you.

Thank you for being who you are and making a world beautiful again.

—Susie Z.
Melbourne
Australia

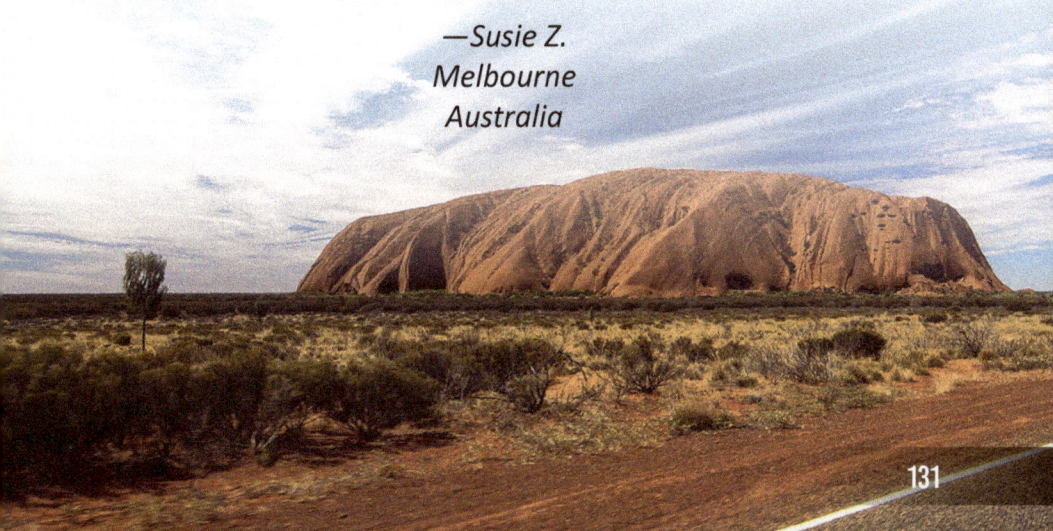

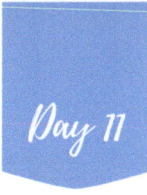

MORNING HUDDLE

Don't Allow the Stress and Pressure of the Day to Cause You to Mentally Tune Out. When You Do So, You Emotionally and Spiritually Go to Sleep.

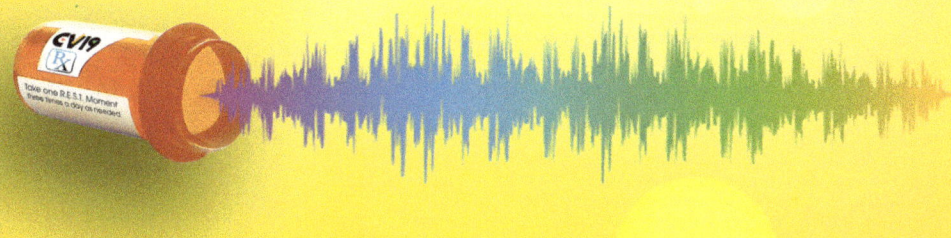

"Wake Up! People need your attention."
—Dr. Chevelta A. Smith

AWAKE

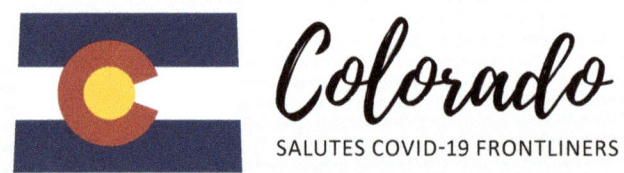

Colorado
SALUTES COVID-19 FRONTLINERS

While the world is debating everything, you wake up and do your job just like every other day. COVID-19 may increase your workload, it may tax your patience, and it may even make you doubt your mission. However, I am here to tell you that I see you. I see you doing what you are called to do. Don't let the world diminish your cause. You were made to face this. You were made to fight this. And while the job may seem overwhelming, your part is greater. Keep your vision straight, and you will be victorious.

—Anne M.
Greeley, Colorado

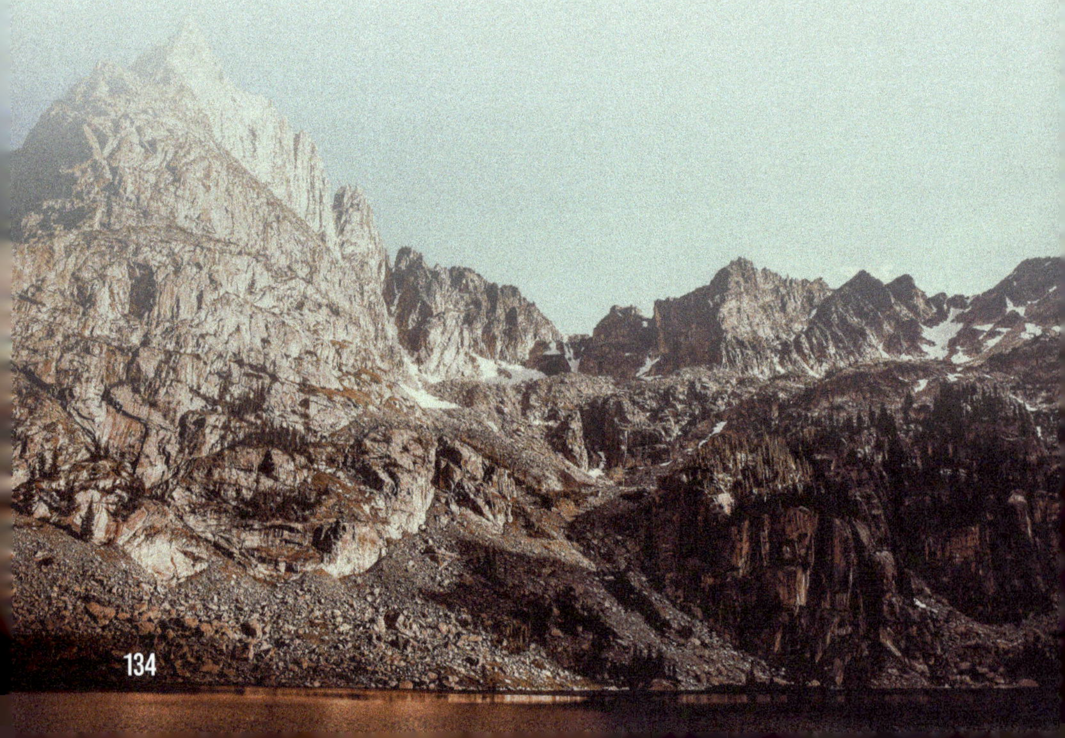

R

Today I RELEASED my... (check all that apply)

Mind By:
- Communicating my thoughts, feelings, & needs to others
- Speaking positive self-affirmations
- Deep breathing
- Other _____

Body By:
- Muscle Relaxation Techniques
- Exercise
- Hydrotherapy: bath or shower
- Other _____

Spirit By:
- Meditation
- Journaling
- Praying
- Going outside for 15-20 minutes
- Self-Talk
- Other _____

E

Today I FEEL... (circle one)

Happy / Anger / Love / Sad / Fear

Surprise / Disgust / Trust / Anticipation

Other _____

What is your dominant EMOTION in your life right now?

S

What were your main STRESSORS today?

What Methods are you using today TO REDUCE your current stress?

What Value have you noticed IN USING them?

T

Stick TOGETHER: How did you Connect today?

- Reached out to a co-worker who appeared to be struggling
- Expressed openly with trusted family or co-workers about how the pandemic is affecting me
- Identified factors that are overwhelming/stressful and worked with others to find solutions
- Initiated the "Buddy" System with other co-workers and monitored each other for signs of stress, burnout, and depression
- Spoke to a mental health care provider

My Let's R.E.S.T. Affirmation for Today:

I am spiritually and emotionally awake so that I may be attentive and sensitive to the needs of others.

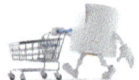
What do you need, but feel like it's unavailable?

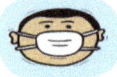
What are you having a hard time expressing?

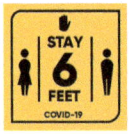
Who or what have you distanced yourself from that could help you overcome the above struggles/difficulties?

NEXT STEPS: Make a healthy plan of action that you will implement in order to help protect yourself from being overtaken by the daily stress of the pandemic. _____
_____
_____
_____
_____
_____
_____

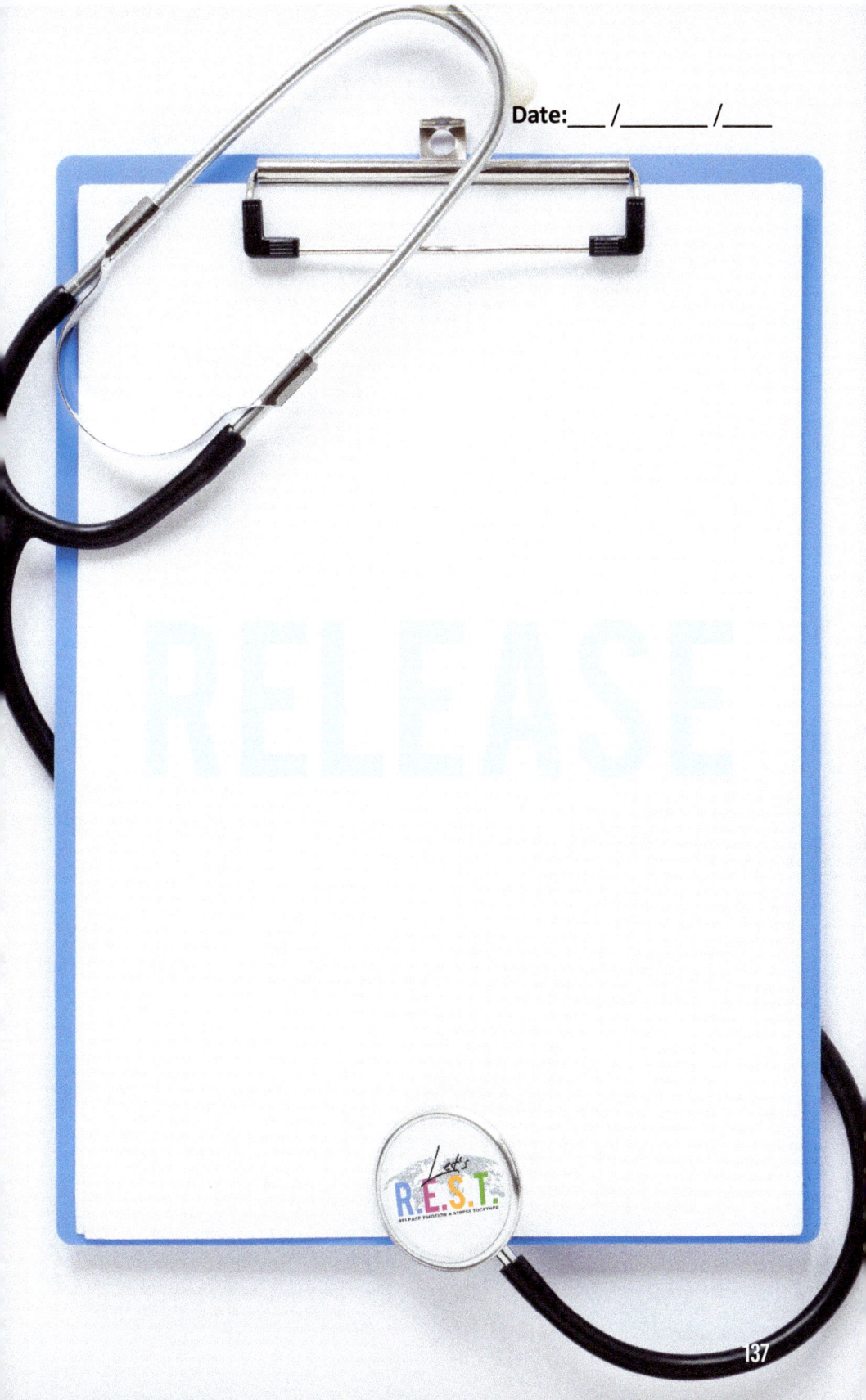

In order to seize our tomorrow, I believe that we must prepare today.
In preparation for tomorrow, I've discovered
that our todays give many lessons.
When we embrace the lessons of today, we are strengthened
emotionally and physically for our tomorrow.
Therefore, the victory for tomorrow is in the submitting to the
inner change and transformation from the lessons of our today.

--Dr. Chevelta A. Smith

> *What* did you learn **TODAY,** and *how* will you apply this knowledge to become a better/healthier you **TOMORROW?**

Let's R.E.S.T. **Bedtime Affirmation**
(Say it out loud!)

I am strong!
I am resilient!
I am able to overcome every disappointment and setback from today
I am more than a conqueror!
I will recharge myself with good sleep tonight
I will awake with a renewed sense of purpose
And I declare that my tomorrow will be great!

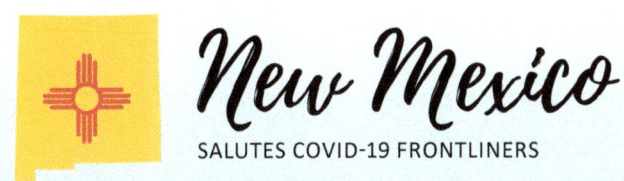

New Mexico
SALUTES COVID-19 FRONTLINERS

Thank you seems too simple and not elaborate enough to express the gratitude we feel for you servicing the community, saving lives, and putting your own lives and your family's lives on the frontline with you.

You have a mission, and God is covering you while you are fighting and protecting others. We are humbled and sincerely grateful. Keep being amazing and stay safe!

*—LaMonica W.
Albuquerque, New Mexico*

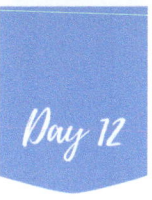
Day 12

MORNING HUDDLE

Move with Intention. Do not Be Distracted. Finish Everything.

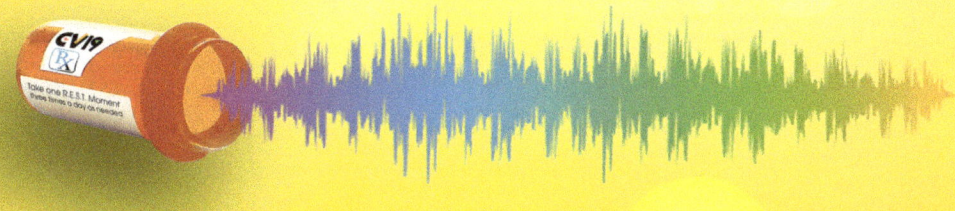

"Be like a lion today—Focus on what your plan of attack will be, in order to accomplish the day with greatness."
—Dr. Chevelta A. Smith

AFFIRMATION FOCUS

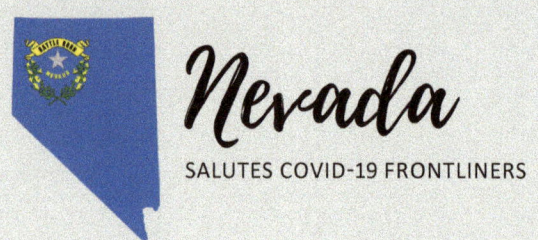

Nevada

SALUTES COVID-19 FRONTLINERS

Fighting with Focus

Thank you for being the warriors that represent the Best of US in this battle of COVID-19. A warrior's most difficult battle will always take place in his heart and mind as he navigates through his core values on a daily basis.

Compassion - Thank you for being led by your heart (that you expose) with every new face you encounter.
Vulnerability - Thank you for showing up every day and giving 100% from the inside out.
Forgiveness - Remembering to forgive the losses and even the lack of support that you may come against.
Focus- Focus on the victories of every life, family, and community that you have impacted by Showing Up!
We Thank You, We Honor You, We Value You, and We Salute YOU!!

Respectfully submitted,
SOS Marriage Network
—Sharon and Oscar Sadler
Henderson, Nevada

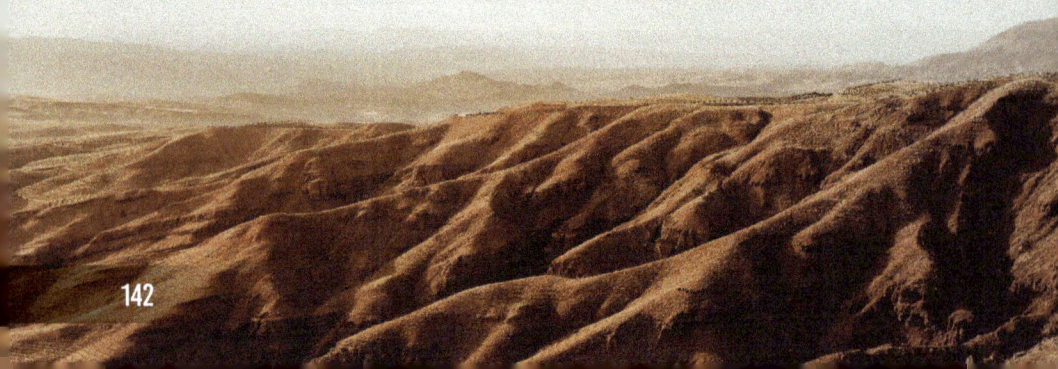

R

Today I RELEASED my... (check all that apply)

Mind By:
- Communicating my thoughts, feelings, & needs to others
- Speaking positive self-affirmations
- Deep breathing
- Other _____

Body By:
- Muscle Relaxation Techniques
- Exercise
- Hydrotherapy: bath or shower
- Other _____

Spirit By:
- Meditation
- Journaling
- Praying
- Going outside for 15-20 minutes
- Self-Talk
- Other _____

E

Today I FEEL... (circle one)

Happy / Anger / Love / Sad / Fear

Surprise / Disgust / Trust / Anticipation

Other _____

What is your dominant **EMOTION** in your life right now?

S

What were your main **STRESSORS** today?

What *Methods* are you using today **TO REDUCE** your current stress?

What *Value* have you noticed **IN USING** them?

T

Stick TOGETHER: How did you *Connect* today?

- Reached out to a co-worker who appeared to be struggling
- Expressed openly with trusted family or co-workers about how the pandemic is affecting me
- Identified factors that are overwhelming/stressful and worked with others to find solutions
- Initiated the "Buddy" System with other co-workers and monitored each other for signs of stress, burnout, and depression
- Spoke to a mental health care provider

My *Let's* R.E.S.T. *Affirmation for Today:*

I am focused! I will not be distracted from what I'm purposed to do today.

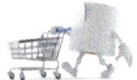 What do you need, but feel like it's unavailable?

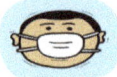 What are you having a hard time expressing?

 Who or what have you distanced yourself from that could help you overcome the above struggles/difficulties?

 **NEXT STEPS:** Make a healthy plan of action that you will implement in order to help protect yourself from being overtaken by the daily stress of the pandemic. _____
_____
_____
_____
_____
_____

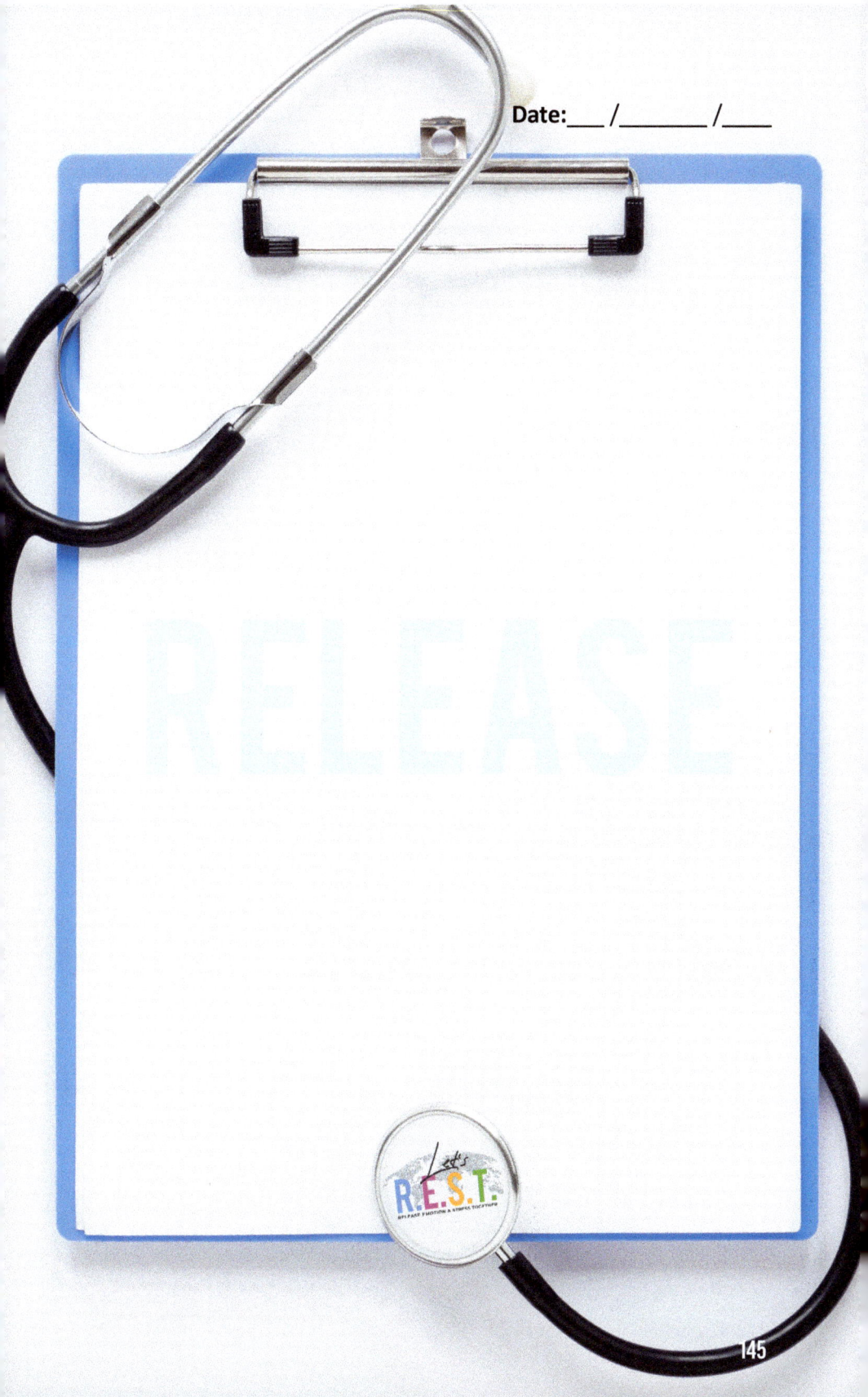

In order to seize our tomorrow, I believe that we must prepare today.
In preparation for tomorrow, I've discovered
that our todays give many lessons.
When we embrace the lessons of today, we are strengthened
emotionally and physically for our tomorrow.
Therefore, the victory for tomorrow is in the submitting to the
inner change and transformation from the lessons of our today.

——Dr. Chevelta A. Smith

What did you learn **TODAY,** and *how* will you apply this knowledge to become a better/healthier you **TOMORROW?**

Let's R.E.S.T. **Bedtime Affirmation**
(Say it out loud!)

I am strong!
I am resilient!
I am able to overcome every disappointment and setback from today
I am more than a conqueror!
I will recharge myself with good sleep tonight
I will awake with a renewed sense of purpose
And I declare that my tomorrow will be great!

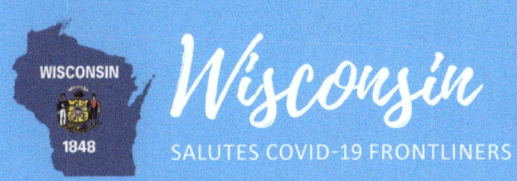

Wisconsin
SALUTES COVID-19 FRONTLINERS

It takes a special person to work the frontlines of this COVID-19. With so many fears, uncertainties, and racial tensions in our society today, it can be very challenging to wonder, is today my turn to be diagnosed. Rather than focus on that, something inside of you says, "I've been trained to make a difference." Though it may not be said much, do know you are loved and appreciated more than you will ever know. Thank you for risking your life just to give a total stranger another chance at life. Thank you for being there, when the families can't, thank you for holding the hands of those who are dying, so they don't die alone.

—Connie R.
Milwaukee, Wisconsin

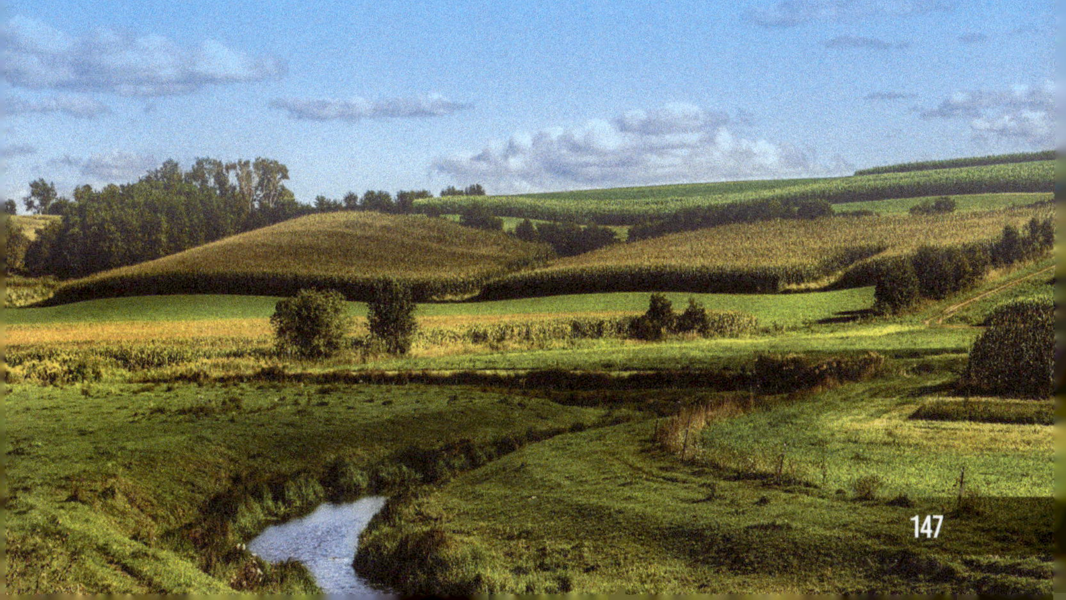

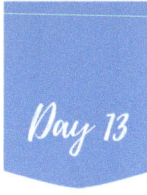

Day 13

MORNING HUDDLE

When You Strengthen Your Mental Immunity…You Will Resist Every Hindrance, Distraction, and Trap That Is Meant to Hold You Back.

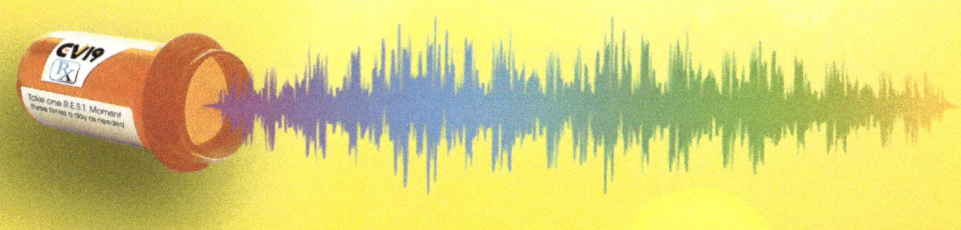

"It's all about your mindset and developing one that is strong!"

—Dr. Chevelta A. Smith

DISTRACTION

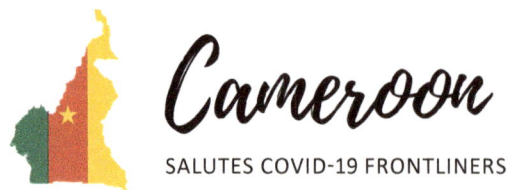

Cameroon

SALUTES COVID-19 FRONTLINERS

To All Our Frontliners

I can't keep calm but shout out a big thank you to you all for working yourselves out every day and especially during this pandemic to rescue humanity. Your dedication is applauded, and your efforts are greatly appreciated. Thank you for your selflessness and relentless efforts. Thank you for putting your lives on the line so that the nations of the world will live to see tomorrow.

Most of you have gone hungry at times, forgoing sleep, rest, and the comfort of your homes & families to respond to our nation's cry for help. No words can express how I personally feel inside about your courage, love, dedication, boldness, efforts, and dedication during this time and beyond. Some of you have died in the process, given your all, yet still squeezing from whatever is left to give. Thank you.

I can only pray that your innermost desires be fulfilled & accomplished. You must have certainly received so many of such messages but know that they come from our hearts, and we mean every word. You are the true heroes of humanity. Only heroes run towards the fight, not away from the fight. To every one of you out there, I say gracias.

—Cera T.
Douala Cameroon
Africa

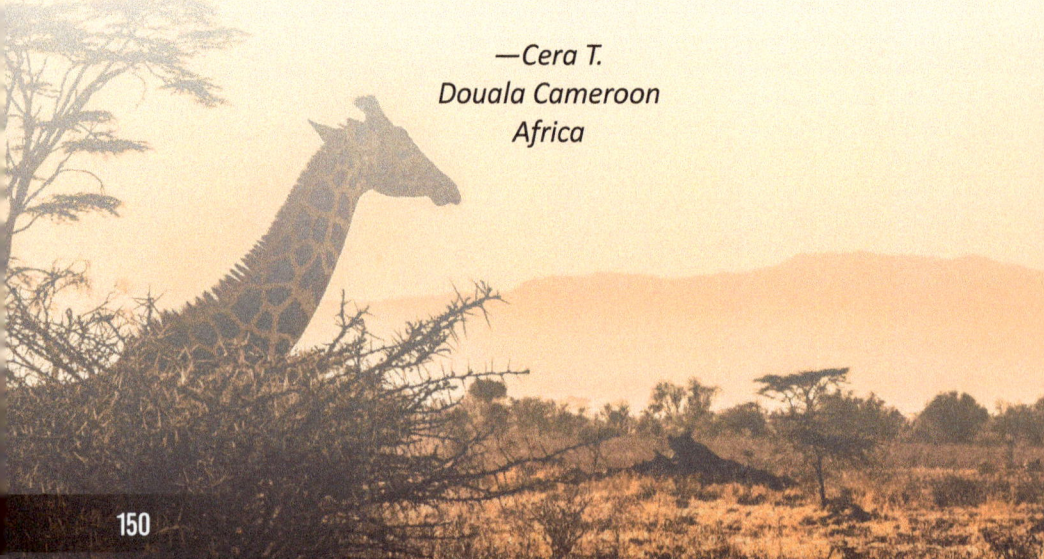

R — Today **I RELEASED** my... (check all that apply)

Mind By:
- Communicating my thoughts, feelings, & needs to others
- Speaking positive self-affirmations
- Deep breathing
- Other _____

Body By:
- Muscle Relaxation Techniques
- Exercise
- Hydrotherapy: bath or shower
- Other _____

Spirit By:
- Meditation
- Journaling
- Praying
- Going outside for 15-20 minutes
- Self-Talk
- Other _____

E — Today **I FEEL**... (circle one)

Happy / Anger / Love / Sad / Fear

Surprise / Disgust / Trust / Anticipation

Other _____

What is your dominant **EMOTION** in your life right now?

S

What were your main **STRESSORS** today?

What *Methods* are you using today **TO REDUCE** your current stress?

What *Value* have you noticed **IN USING** them?

T — Stick **TOGETHER**: How did you *Connect* today?

- Reached out to a co-worker who appeared to be struggling
- Expressed openly with trusted family or co-workers about how the pandemic is affecting me
- Identified factors that are overwhelming/stressful and worked with others to find solutions
- Initiated the "Buddy" System with other co-workers and monitored each other for signs of stress, burnout, and depression
- Spoke to a mental health care provider

My *Let's* R.E.S.T. *Affirmation for Today:*

I will fix my attention on the things that are important for me to accomplish today. I will avoid distractions that can hinder my ability to perform with excellence.

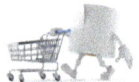
What do you need, but feel like it's unavailable?

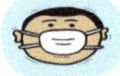
What are you having a hard time expressing?

Who or what have you distanced yourself from that could help you overcome the above struggles/difficulties?

NEXT STEPS: Make a healthy plan of action that you will implement in order to help protect yourself from being overtaken by the daily stress of the pandemic. _____
_____
_____
_____
_____
_____
_____

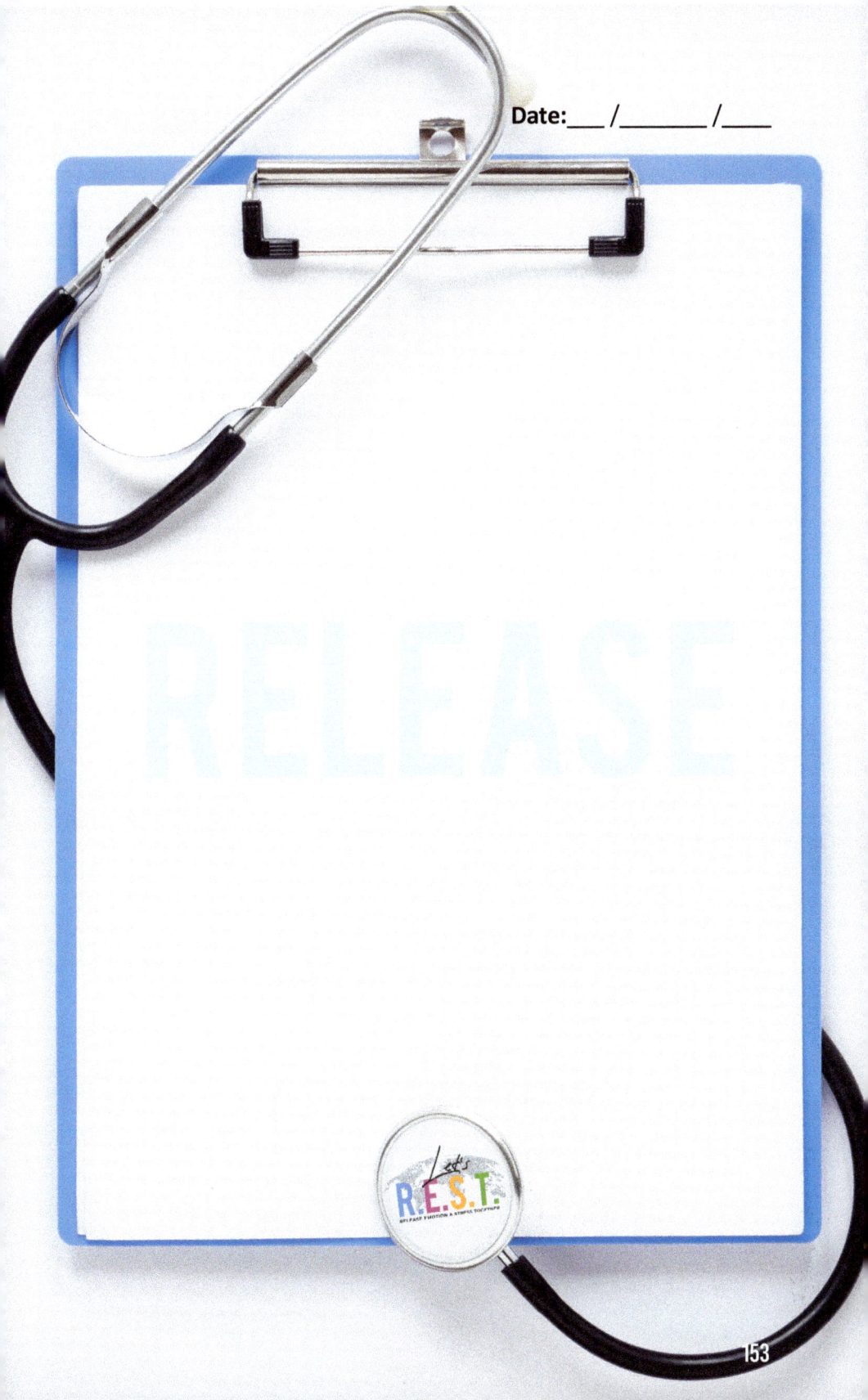

In order to seize our tomorrow, I believe that we must prepare today.
In preparation for tomorrow, I've discovered
that our todays give many lessons.
When we embrace the lessons of today, we are strengthened
emotionally and physically for our tomorrow.
Therefore, the victory for tomorrow is in the submitting to the
inner change and transformation from the lessons of our today.

—–Dr. Chevelta A. Smith

What did you learn **TODAY**, and *how* will you apply this knowledge to become a better/healthier you **TOMORROW?**

Let's R.E.S.T. **Bedtime Affirmation**
(Say it out loud!)

I am strong!
I am resilient!
I am able to overcome every disappointment and setback from today
I am more than a conqueror!
I will recharge myself with good sleep tonight
I will awake with a renewed sense of purpose
And I declare that my tomorrow will be great!

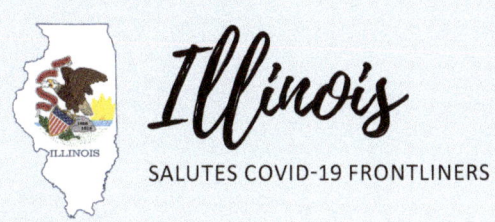

Illinois
SALUTES COVID-19 FRONTLINERS

To All: COVID-19 Medical Frontliners
I would like to take this time to let you all know how much you are loved and appreciated!

From your family in Chicago, IL, you all are constantly in our thoughts and prayers. God Bless!

—Derek E.
Chicago, Illinois

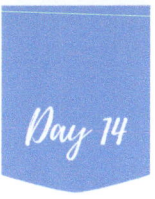

Day 14

MORNING HUDDLE

We Have to Get Into the Practice of Assessing Ourselves and Making Sure that We are Okay.

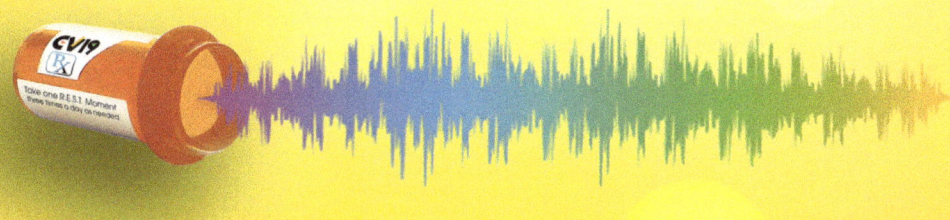

"Excuse me! I'm in an appointment with myself."
—Dr. Chevelta A. Smith

ASSESS

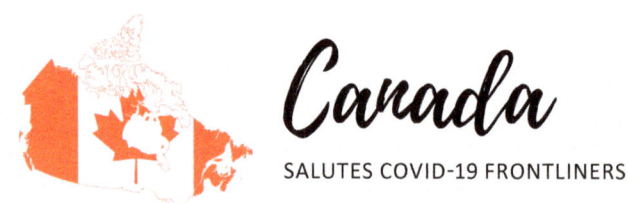

Canada

SALUTES COVID-19 FRONTLINERS

Every day, as I watch the news, I am continually proud and grateful for the tireless work that all our frontline workers accomplish -- Sacrificing time with their families, friends, loved ones, and, putting themselves directly in the face of danger while maintaining their pledge to serve the community. You are our superheroes! We know you're exhausted and extremely overwhelmed but know we are praying for your continued spiritual, physical, and mental health! When all of this is over and under control, you must take pride in knowing your fight against this pandemic will be recorded in the pages of history, and because of your commitment, WE SURVIVED!
God bless you all!

—Dayle J.
Toronto, Ontario Canada

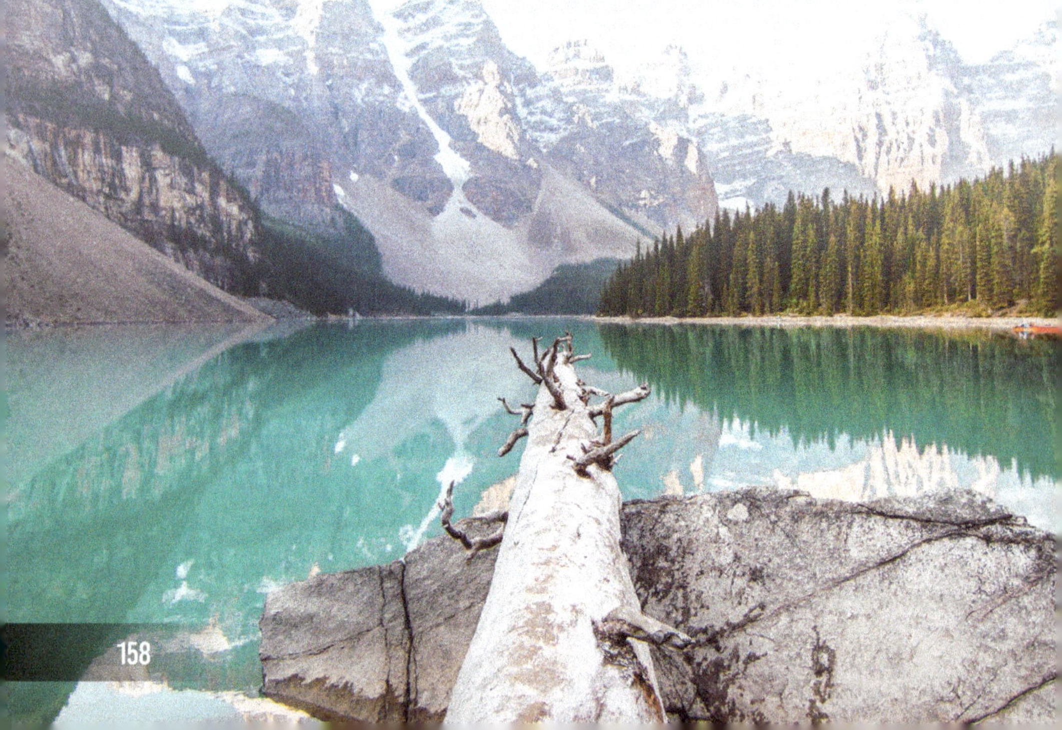

R — Today I RELEASED my... (check all that apply)

Mind By:
- Communicating my thoughts, feelings, & needs to others
- Speaking positive self-affirmations
- Deep breathing
- Other _____

Body By:
- Muscle Relaxation Techniques
- Exercise
- Hydrotherapy: bath or shower
- Other _____

Spirit By:
- Meditation
- Journaling
- Praying
- Going outside for 15-20 minutes
- Self-Talk
- Other _____

E — Today I FEEL... (circle one)

Happy / Anger / Love / Sad / Fear

Surprise / Disgust / Trust / Anticipation

Other _____

What is your dominant **EMOTION** in your life right now?

S

What were your main **STRESSORS** today?

What *Methods* are you using today **TO REDUCE** your current stress?

What *Value* have you noticed **IN USING** them?

T — Stick TOGETHER: How did you *Connect* today?

- Reached out to a co-worker who appeared to be struggling
- Expressed openly with trusted family or co-workers about how the pandemic is affecting me
- Identified factors that are overwhelming/stressful and worked with others to find solutions
- Initiated the "Buddy" System with other co-workers and monitored each other for signs of stress, burnout, and depression
- Spoke to a mental health care provider

My ~~Let's~~ R.E.S.T. *Affirmation for Today:*

I will examine myself honestly today. I will seek help or treatment where it's needed. I am restoring my body, soul, and spirit so that I can be whole and healthy.

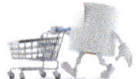 What do you need, but feel like it's unavailable?

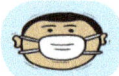 What are you having a hard time expressing?

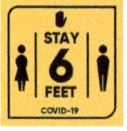 Who or what have you distanced yourself from that could help you overcome the above struggles/difficulties?

 **NEXT STEPS:** Make a healthy plan of action that you will implement in order to help protect yourself from being overtaken by the daily stress of the pandemic. _____
_____
_____
_____
_____
_____
_____

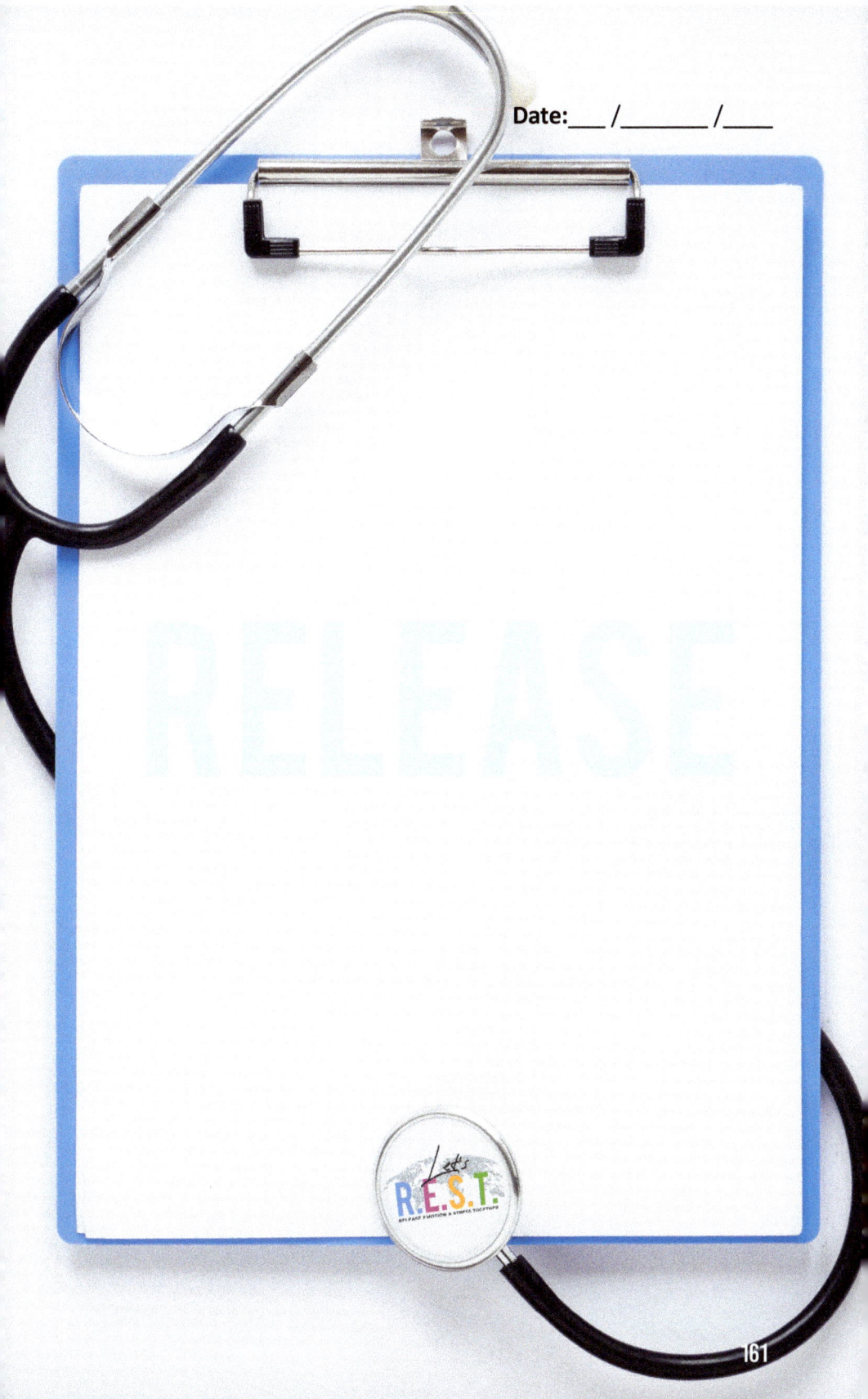

In order to seize our tomorrow, I believe that we must prepare today.
In preparation for tomorrow, I've discovered
that our todays give many lessons.
When we embrace the lessons of today, we are strengthened
emotionally and physically for our tomorrow.
Therefore, the victory for tomorrow is in the submitting to the
inner change and transformation from the lessons of our today.

– – Dr. Chevelta A. Smith

What did you learn **TODAY**, and *how* will you apply this knowledge to become a better/healthier you **TOMORROW?**

Let's R.E.S.T. **Bedtime Affirmation**
(Say it out loud!)

I am strong!
I am resilient!
I am able to overcome every disappointment and setback from today
I am more than a conqueror!
I will recharge myself with good sleep tonight
I will awake with a renewed sense of purpose
And I declare that my tomorrow will be great!

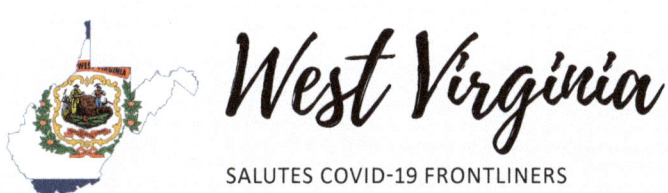

West Virginia

SALUTES COVID-19 FRONTLINERS

To all of the nurses working on the frontlines during this pandemic, THANK YOU! I know that what you have been doing from the start of this, what you are currently doing, and what you will continue to do during this pandemic is hard work, disheartening at times, and shattering you every day as you watch someone else die without a loved one present. I appreciate all of your work, effort, and kindness that you show to people during this pandemic. May we all be comforted by nurses as hardworking and as caring as you during this time, THANK YOU for everything and all of the sacrifices you are making to do this job while keeping your families safe.

—Erica H.
West Virginia

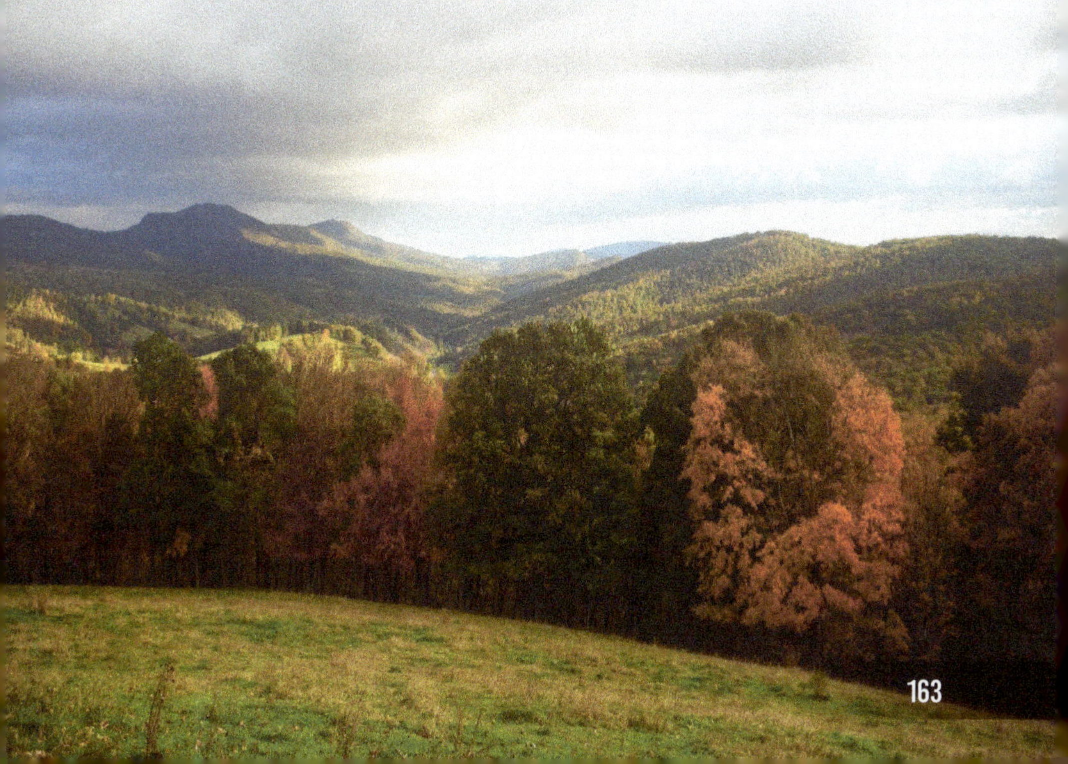

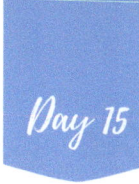

Day 15

MORNING HUDDLE

It's Important That You Do Not Quit! Continue to Be Consistent and Persistent in All that You Are Striving to Achieve. You Are Destined to Finish Everything You've Started With Excellence.

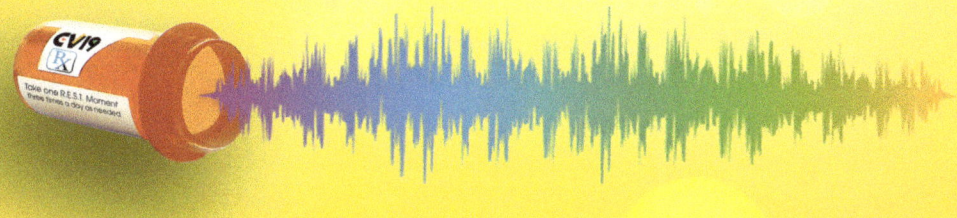

"Don't be present but missing in life. Persist to exist, Exist to live."

—Dr. Chevelta A. Smith

PERSISTENCE

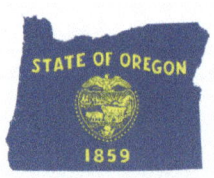

Oregon

SALUTES COVID-19 FRONTLINERS

During the first weeks of the pandemic, patients were filling your offices and emergency rooms with an unknown outcome, yet you were brave. As the general public refused to believe COVID-19 was real, you persisted with your responsibilities to treat patients who were living and dying proof of this virus. Each new day presented you with countless opportunities to walk away, to protect yourselves and your families. Yet, you spent unprecedented hours caring for those who were infected. With no outside support, you became the family, the friends, the support group, and the mourners for the patients who were suddenly found isolated from the world. For some, you were the last person they saw before they succumbed to the virus.

You continue to persist still today. Even as the numbers continue to rise, despite countless expert warnings to 'slow the spread' --you do not stop providing care. From the depth of my soul, I thank you for never faltering on your oath. From the medical experts to the medical cleanup crew, you are genuine heroes. The world is a better place because of your selflessness.

—Dr. Monica Beane
Salem, Oregon

R — Today **I RELEASED** *my*... (check all that apply)

Mind By:
- Communicating my thoughts, feelings, & needs to others
- Speaking positive self-affirmations
- Deep breathing
- Other _____

Body By:
- Muscle Relaxation Techniques
- Exercise
- Hydrotherapy: bath or shower
- Other _____

Spirit By:
- Meditation
- Journaling
- Praying
- Going outside for 15-20 minutes
- Self-Talk
- Other _____

E — Today **I FEEL**... *(circle one)*

Happy / Anger / Love / Sad / Fear

Surprise / Disgust / Trust / Anticipation

Other _____

What is your dominant **EMOTION** in your life right now?

S

What were your main **STRESSORS** today?

What *Methods* are you using today **TO REDUCE** your current stress?

What *Value* have you noticed **IN USING** them?

T — Stick **TOGETHER**: How did you *Connect* today?

- Reached out to a co-worker who appeared to be struggling
- Expressed openly with trusted family or co-workers about how the pandemic is affecting me
- Identified factors that are overwhelming/stressful and worked with others to find solutions
- Initiated the "Buddy" System with other co-workers and monitored each other for signs of stress, burnout, and depression
- Spoke to a mental health care provider

My *Let's* **R.E.S.T.** *Affirmation for Today:*

I will not grow weary in doing good during this pandemic. I will persevere on my job even when I'm tired or frustrated. I will not give up!

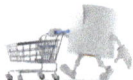
What do you need, but feel like it's unavailable?

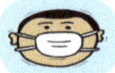
What are you having a hard time expressing?

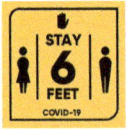
Who or what have you distanced yourself from that could help you overcome the above struggles/difficulties?

NEXT STEPS: Make a healthy plan of action that you will implement in order to help protect yourself from being overtaken by the daily stress of the pandemic. _____
_____
_____
_____
_____
_____
_____

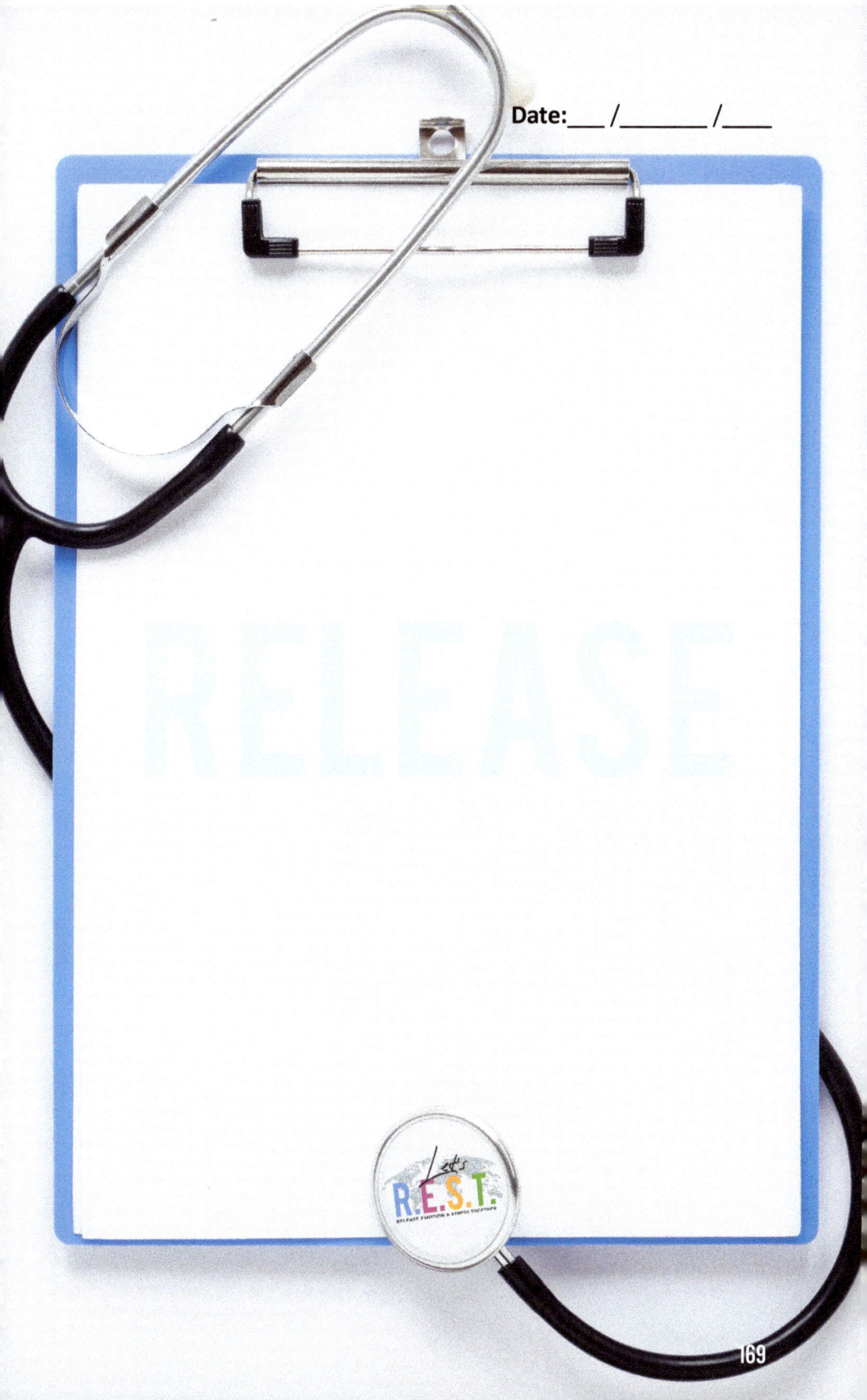

In order to seize our tomorrow, I believe that we must prepare today.
In preparation for tomorrow, I've discovered
that our todays give many lessons.
When we embrace the lessons of today, we are strengthened
emotionally and physically for our tomorrow.
Therefore, the victory for tomorrow is in the submitting to the
inner change and transformation from the lessons of our today.

--Dr. Chevelta A. Smith

What did you learn **TODAY,** and *how* will you apply this knowledge to become a better/healthier you **TOMORROW?**

Let's R.E.S.T. **Bedtime Affirmation**
(Say it out loud!)

I am strong!
I am resilient!
I am able to overcome every disappointment and setback from today
I am more than a conqueror!
I will recharge myself with good sleep tonight
I will awake with a renewed sense of purpose
And I declare that my tomorrow will be great!

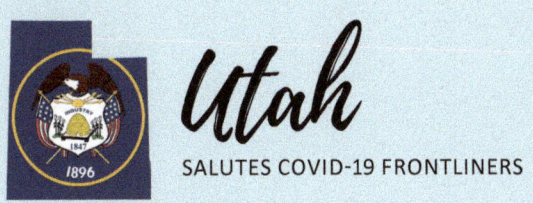

Utah
SALUTES COVID-19 FRONTLINERS

As we drove up to the clinic, I could see that they were ready. A man at the entrance to the parking lot was waiting. He told us which spot to park in, and then a clinic worker immediately came to the car window. She asked me a few questions and took my cell phone number. I would receive a call in a few minutes, she said. When the call came, we were told to drive around to the tent. A woman in full PPE explained the procedure and swabbed my right nostril. Within 48 hours, I had my test results. Negative. I was relieved and grateful to these frontline workers who took such care, who take such care with every person who needs them. Day after day, they persist. They care. To them, and to all the medical workers, I am grateful.

—Sylvia R.
Logan, Utah

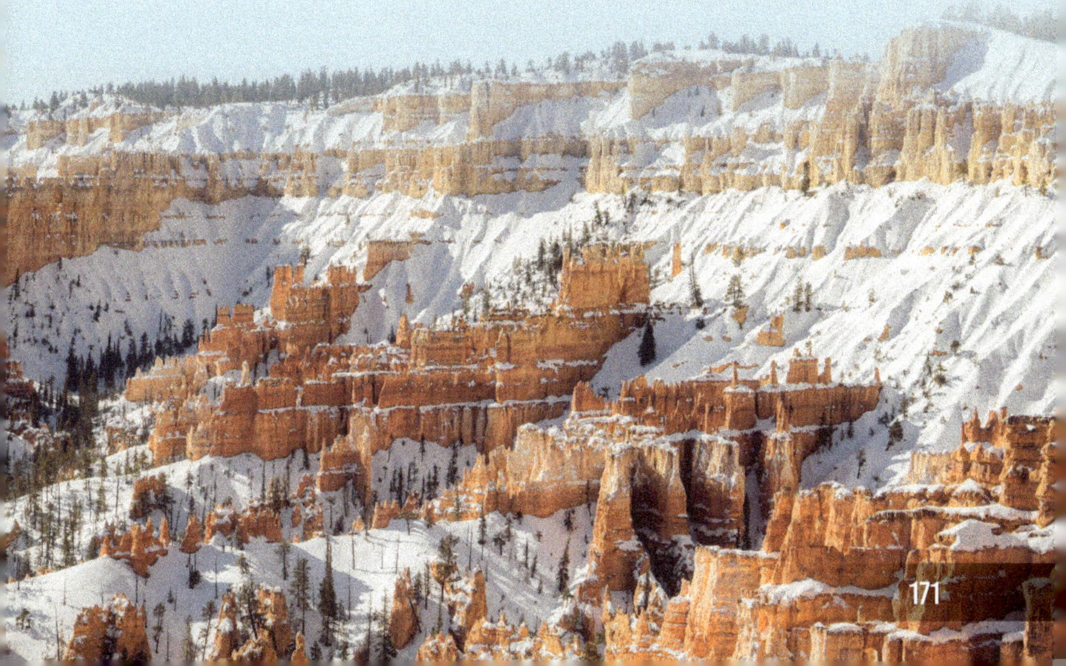

Let's R.E.S.T. **CHECK POINT**

You are half way through the *Let's* R.E.S.T. Morning Huddles. This is a great time to STOP and ASSESS how are you doing.

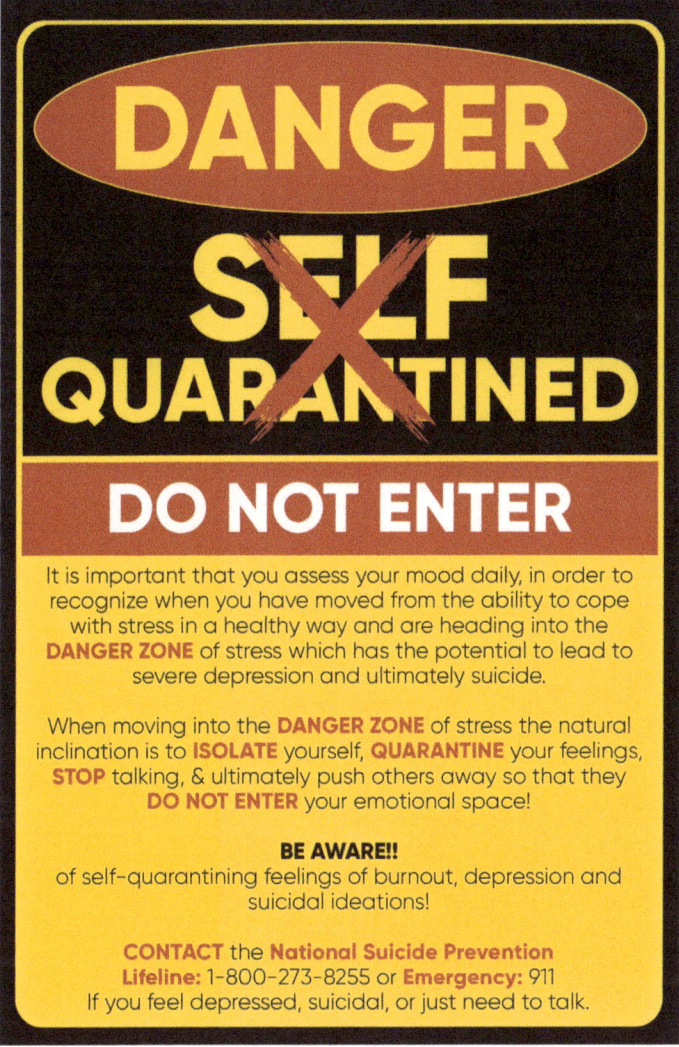

Throughout the remainder of this *Let's* R.E.S.T. Journal, continue to track your mood and assess whether you are heading into or have entered the DANGER Zone of stress & burnout!

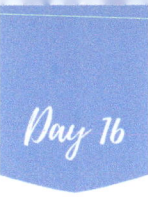

Day 16

MORNING HUDDLE

You Are Worthy of Happiness. You Are Worthy of Success. You Are Worthy of Love and Peace, and You Are Worthy of Appreciation.

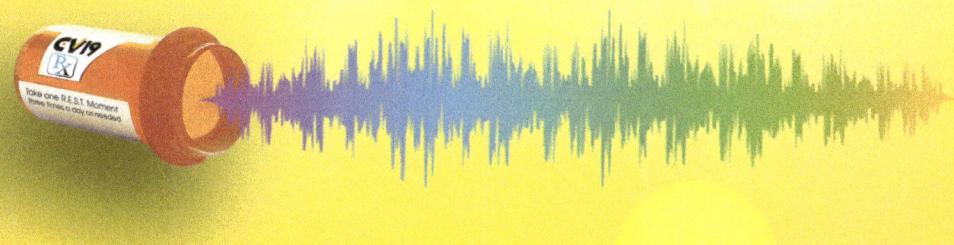

"Think of all the good things you've been waiting to come your way. Now, open your heart to receive them."
—Dr. Chevelta A. Smith

AFFIRMATION WORTHY

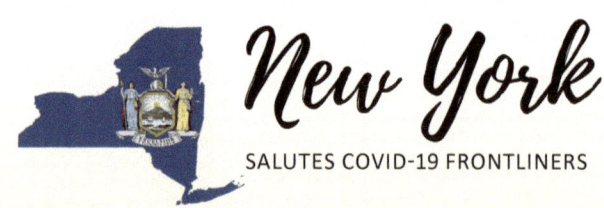

New York
SALUTES COVID-19 FRONTLINERS

Living in the heart of NYC in the spring, we had a lot of bad news and reasons to feel scared and insecure but, every night at 7 pm, we had hope and optimism as we remembered our frontline workers holding the line and saving lives. It seemed, with each passing day, cheers grew louder, pounding stronger, and beating drums multiplied. We clapped our hands sore from every window, rooftops and the streets around us. The cheers echoed in the steel and concrete canyons of New York. Our hearts turned each night to our heroes nearby by not only saving lives but providing inspiration. God bless the frontline workers and keep them strong and safe.

*—Kyle B.
Manhattan, New York*

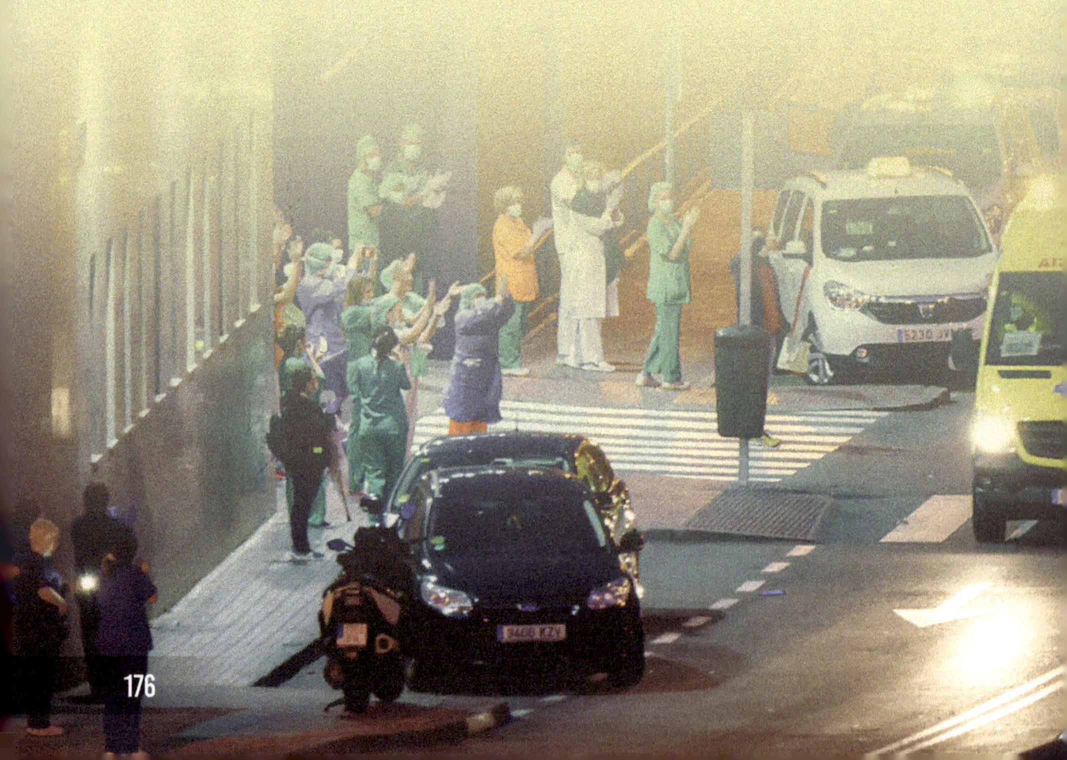

R

Today I RELEASED my... (check all that apply)

Mind By:
- Communicating my thoughts, feelings, & needs to others
- Speaking positive self-affirmations
- Deep breathing
- Other _____

Body By:
- Muscle Relaxation Techniques
- Exercise
- Hydrotherapy: bath or shower
- Other _____

Spirit By:
- Meditation
- Journaling
- Praying
- Going outside for 15-20 minutes
- Self-Talk
- Other _____

E

Today I FEEL... (circle one)

Happy / Anger / Love / Sad / Fear

Surprise / Disgust / Trust / Anticipation

Other _____

What is your dominant **EMOTION** in your life right now?

S

What were your main **STRESSORS** today?

What *Methods* are you using today **TO REDUCE** your current stress?

What *Value* have you noticed **IN USING** them?

T

Stick TOGETHER: How did you *Connect* today?

- Reached out to a co-worker who appeared to be struggling
- Expressed openly with trusted family or co-workers about how the pandemic is affecting me
- Identified factors that are overwhelming/stressful and worked with others to find solutions
- Initiated the "Buddy" System with other co-workers and monitored each other for signs of stress, burnout, and depression
- Spoke to a mental health care provider

My Let's R.E.S.T. Affirmation for Today:
I am worthy of love. I am worthy of appreciation. I am worthy of success

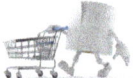 What do you need, but feel like it's unavailable?

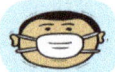 What are you having a hard time expressing?

 Who or what have you distanced yourself from that could help you overcome the above struggles/difficulties?

 **NEXT STEPS:** Make a healthy plan of action that you will implement in order to help protect yourself from being overtaken by the daily stress of the pandemic. _____
_____
_____
_____
_____
_____

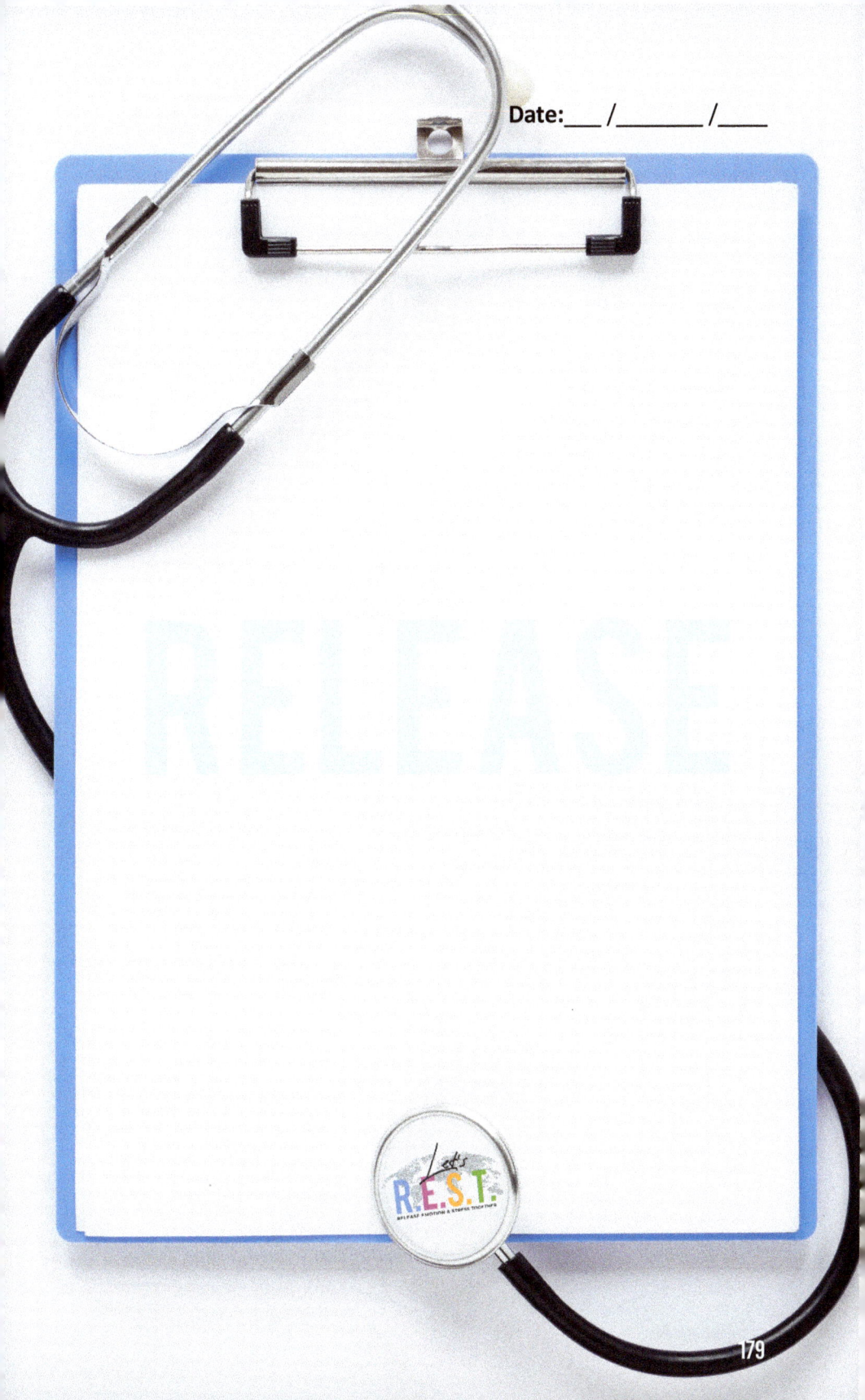

Date:___ / _____ / ___

RELEASE

In order to seize our tomorrow, I believe that we must prepare today.
In preparation for tomorrow, I've discovered
that our todays give many lessons.
When we embrace the lessons of today, we are strengthened
emotionally and physically for our tomorrow.
Therefore, the victory for tomorrow is in the submitting to the
inner change and transformation from the lessons of our today.

— — Dr. Chevelta A. Smith

> *What* did you learn **TODAY,** and *how* will you apply this knowledge to become a better/healthier you **TOMORROW?**

Let's R.E.S.T. Bedtime Affirmation
(Say it out loud!)

I am strong!
I am resilient!
I am able to overcome every disappointment and setback from today
I am more than a conqueror!
I will recharge myself with good sleep tonight
I will awake with a renewed sense of purpose
And I declare that my tomorrow will be great!

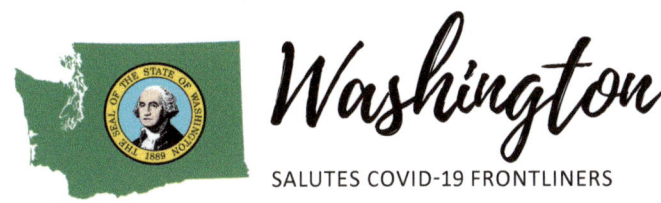

Washington
SALUTES COVID-19 FRONTLINERS

We don't often see that there is a backbone that supports our community, a pillar of support that comprises unseen people and overlooked functions. One such pillar in these times of a global pandemic is: our health professionals who are working without recognition to save the lives of those who are falling victim to this disease. Without them, we would be far worse off, and there would be fewer people who recovered from the ravages of this epidemic. Often serving away from the glare of publicity, these people dive into the most extreme cases and the direst situations, doing the best they can for each patient, diligently observing their oath to save the lives of those who are under their care.

These frontline professionals do not risk their lives unwillingly or cheaply. They know the risks of their own infection by this disease, and they know the prognosis is often grim even for the most, well-educated and well-protected individual who gets sick. Still, they go to work, doing their duty, to a population that sometimes does not acknowledge their risk. But we do recognize them and thank them for their service.

Thank you,
—Stephen Matlock
North Bend, Washington

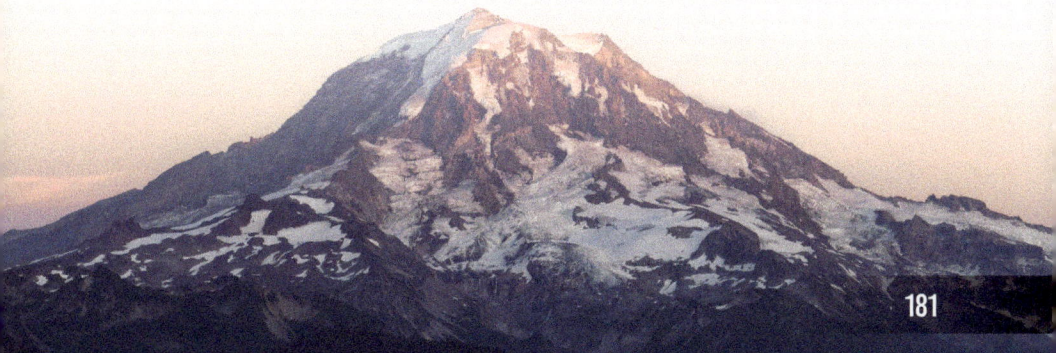

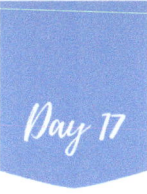

Day 17

MORNING HUDDLE

Your Mind and How You Think Will Determine How You Will Succeed in Life. Resist Fear. Become Immune to the Stinking Thinking That Tells You You're Not Good Enough.

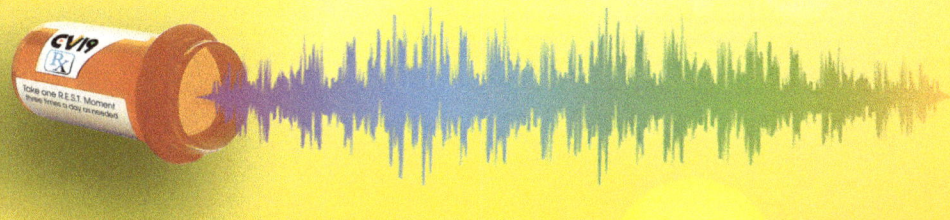

"Life can't be controlled, but my response to it can!"
—Dr. Chevelta A. Smith

IMMUNITY

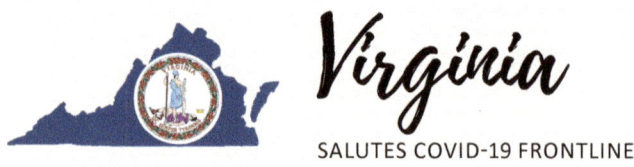

Virginia

SALUTES COVID-19 FRONTLINERS

I can't imagine the stress and frustration you may feel on any given day, but I can appreciate your heroism and the sacrifice you consistently make to care for patients who are sick, fearful, and fighting for their lives. Your devotion, expertise, improvisation, and service beyond the call of duty give family members hope and a boost of confidence in what would otherwise be unsure, lonely, and obscured situations.

Thank you for your assistance. It is not taken for granted that you are putting your lives on the line for strangers. Take courage. There is a beautiful passage recorded in the Holy Bible that states, "When I am weak, I am strong for God's Grace is sufficient for me." You have certainly proven your strength and courage.

—*Pastor Ivory Bostick*
Springfield, Virginia

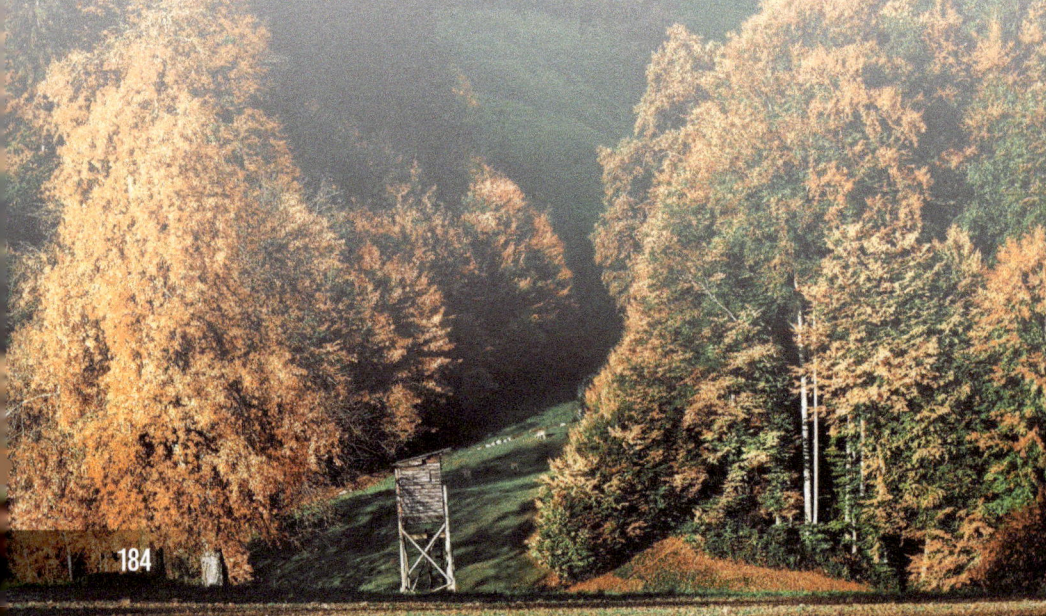

R

Today I RELEASED my... *(check all that apply)*

Mind By:
- Communicating my thoughts, feelings, & needs to others
- Speaking positive self-affirmations ■ Deep breathing ■ Other _____

Body By:
- Muscle Relaxation Techniques   ■ Exercise
- Hydrotherapy: bath or shower   ■ Other _____

Spirit By:
- Meditation   ■ Journaling   ■ Praying
- Going outside for 15-20 minutes   ■ Self-Talk   ■ Other _____

E

Today I FEEL... *(circle one)*

Happy / Anger / Love / Sad / Fear

Surprise / Disgust / Trust / Anticipation

*Other*_____

What is your dominant **EMOTION** in your life right now?

S

What were your main **STRESSORS** today?

What *Methods* are you using today **TO REDUCE** your current stress?

What *Value* have you noticed **IN USING** them?

T

Stick TOGETHER: How did you *Connect* today?

- Reached out to a co-worker who appeared to be struggling
- Expressed openly with trusted family or co-workers about how the pandemic is affecting me
- Identified factors that are overwhelming/stressful and worked with others to find solutions
- Initiated the "Buddy" System with other co-workers and monitored each other for signs of stress, burnout, and depression
- Spoke to a mental health care provider

My Let's R.E.S.T. Affirmation for Today:
I will resist negative thoughts about myself. I am enough. I am a masterpiece.

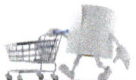 What do you need, but feel like it's unavailable?

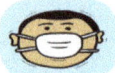 What are you having a hard time expressing?

 Who or what have you distanced yourself from that could help you overcome the above struggles/difficulties?

 **NEXT STEPS:** Make a healthy plan of action that you will implement in order to help protect yourself from being overtaken by the daily stress of the pandemic. _____
_____
_____
_____
_____
_____
_____

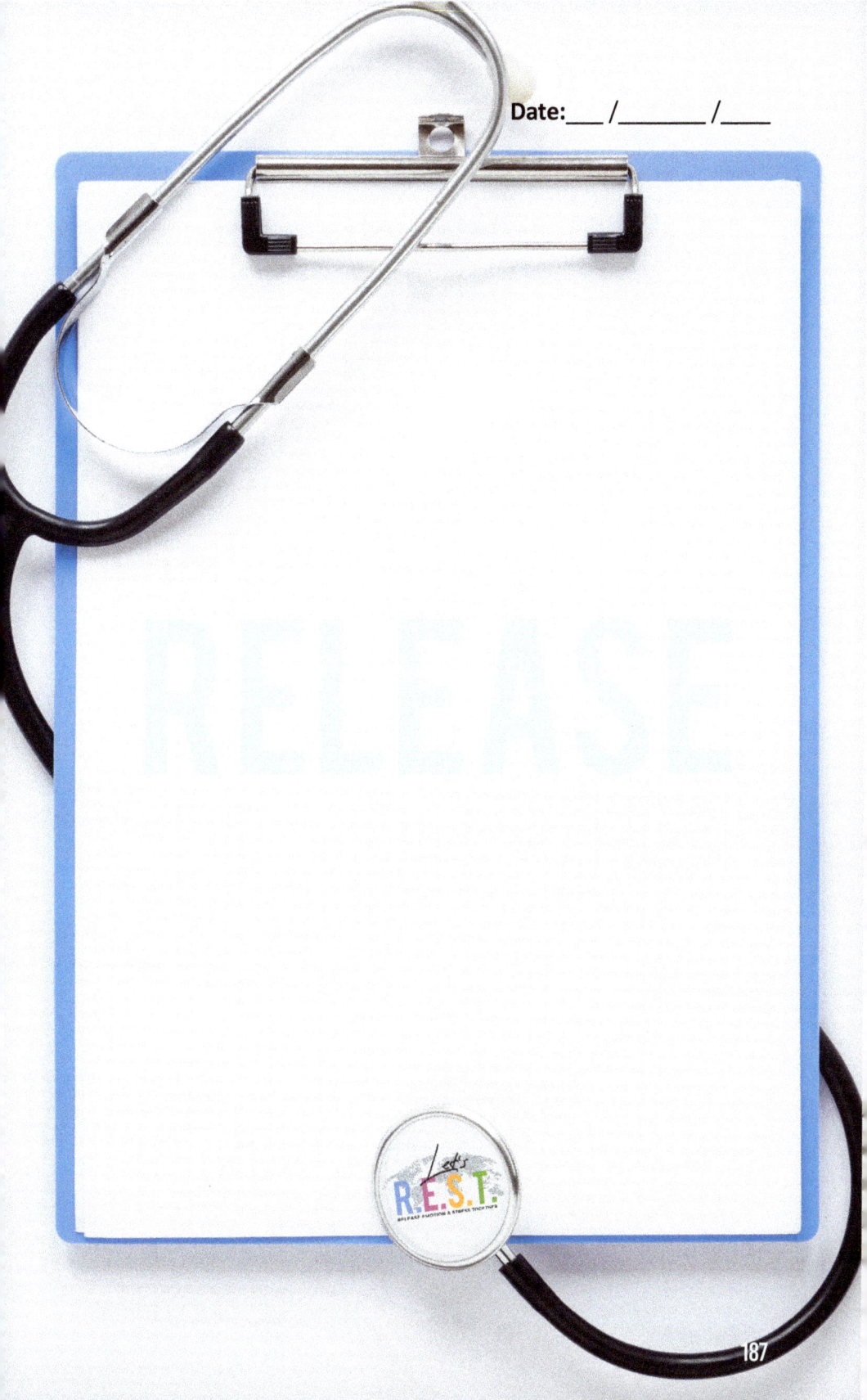

In order to seize our tomorrow, I believe that we must prepare today.
In preparation for tomorrow, I've discovered
that our todays give many lessons.
When we embrace the lessons of today, we are strengthened
emotionally and physically for our tomorrow.
Therefore, the victory for tomorrow is in the submitting to the
inner change and transformation from the lessons of our today.

—–Dr. Chevelta A. Smith

What did you learn **TODAY,** and *how* will you apply this knowledge to become a better/healthier you **TOMORROW?**

Let's R.E.S.T. **Bedtime Affirmation**
(Say it out loud!)

I am strong!
I am resilient!
I am able to overcome every disappointment and setback from today
I am more than a conqueror!
I will recharge myself with good sleep tonight
I will awake with a renewed sense of purpose
And I declare that my tomorrow will be great!

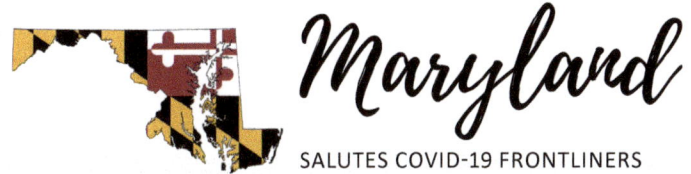

Maryland
SALUTES COVID-19 FRONTLINERS

I want to take a moment just to say how much I admire and appreciate your consistent dedication and commitment. You continue to serve those that you may have never met or will ever see again...but yet you continue to provide top-notch and outstanding services every day. Thanks for ALL you do, and please be safe.

—Joyce J.
Edgewood, Maryland

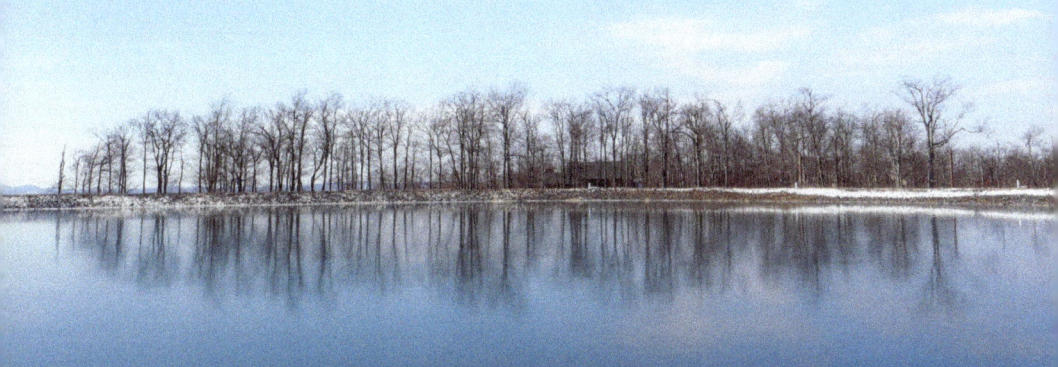

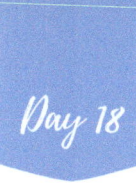

Day 18

MORNING HUDDLE

As You Go Through Life, You Will Continue to Discover the Greatness That's in You.

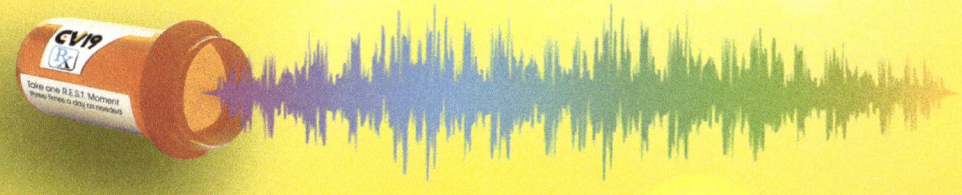

"If we are ever learning, then we will always continue to be ever growing."

—Dr. Chevelta A. Smith

DISCOVER

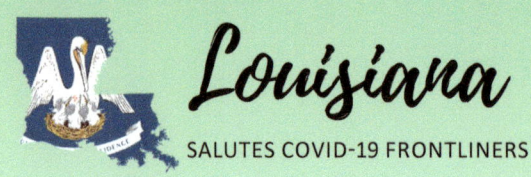

Louisiana

SALUTES COVID-19 FRONTLINERS

We never knew this time would be so disastrous. We never knew how important your service would be needed. Just know your unselfish love, hard work, and dedication during this pandemic will never be forgotten and will forever be in the hearts of the American people.

—*Sonja S.*
Baton Rouge, Louisiana

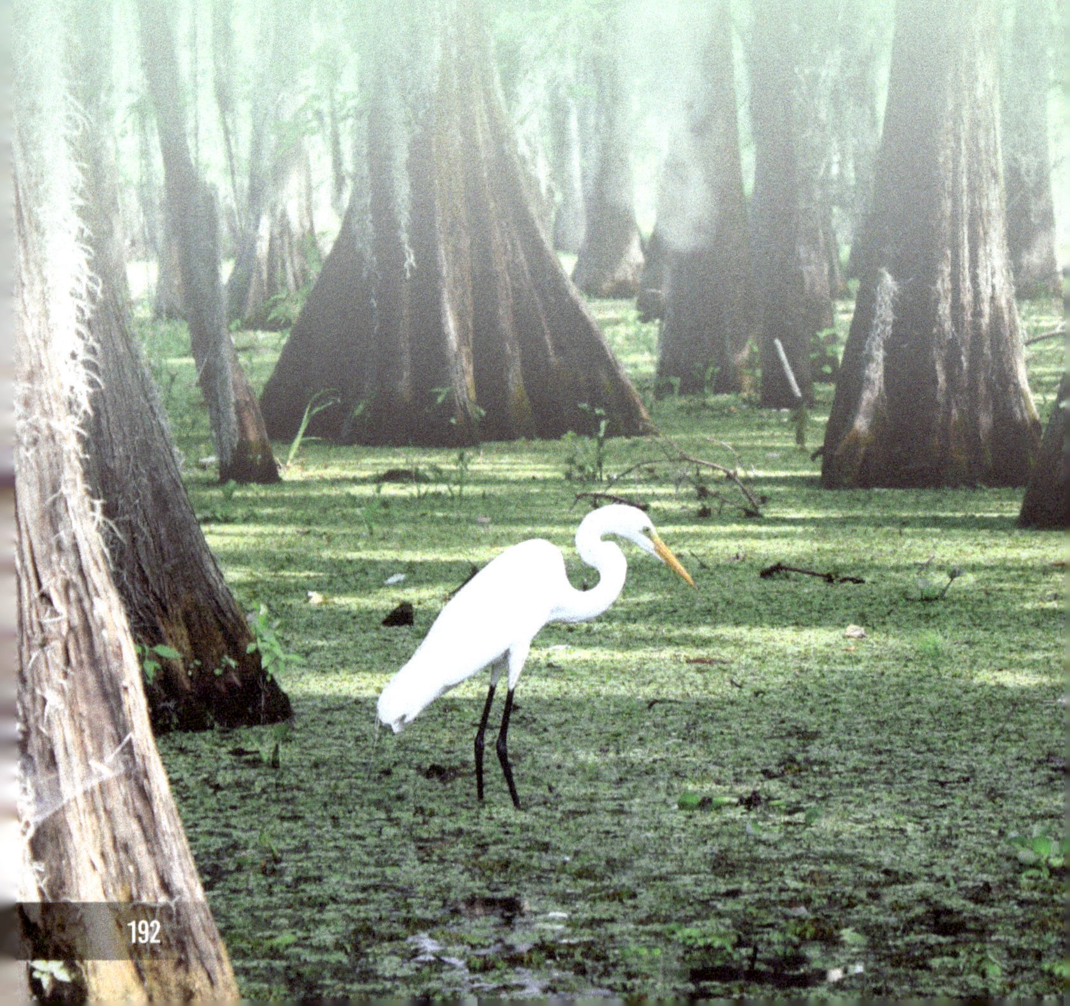

R — Today I RELEASED my... (check all that apply)

Mind By:
- ☐ Communicating my thoughts, feelings, & needs to others
- ☐ Speaking positive self-affirmations   ☐ Deep breathing   ☐ Other _____

Body By:
- ☐ Muscle Relaxation Techniques   ☐ Exercise
- ☐ Hydrotherapy: bath or shower   ☐ Other _____

Spirit By:
- ☐ Meditation   ☐ Journaling   ☐ Praying
- ☐ Going outside for 15-20 minutes   ☐ Self-Talk   ☐ Other _____

E — Today I FEEL... (circle one)

Happy / Anger / Love / Sad / Fear

Surprise / Disgust / Trust / Anticipation

Other_____

What is your dominant **EMOTION** in your life right now?

S

What were your main **STRESSORS** today?

What *Methods* are you using today **TO REDUCE** your current stress?

What *Value* have you noticed **IN USING** them?

T — Stick TOGETHER: How did you *Connect* today?

- Reached out to a co-worker who appeared to be struggling
- Expressed openly with trusted family or co-workers about how the pandemic is affecting me
- Identified factors that are overwhelming/stressful and worked with others to find solutions
- Initiated the "Buddy" System with other co-workers and monitored each other for signs of stress, burnout, and depression
- Spoke to a mental health care provider

My *Let's* R.E.S.T. Affirmation for Today:
I am discovering the greatness within me. I am filled with wonderful gifts and talents.

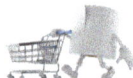 What do you need, but feel like it's unavailable?

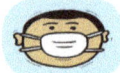 What are you having a hard time expressing?

 Who or what have you distanced yourself from that could help you overcome the above struggles/difficulties?

 **NEXT STEPS: Make a healthy plan of action that you will implement in order to help protect yourself from being overtaken by the daily stress of the pandemic.** _____
_____
_____
_____
_____
_____
_____

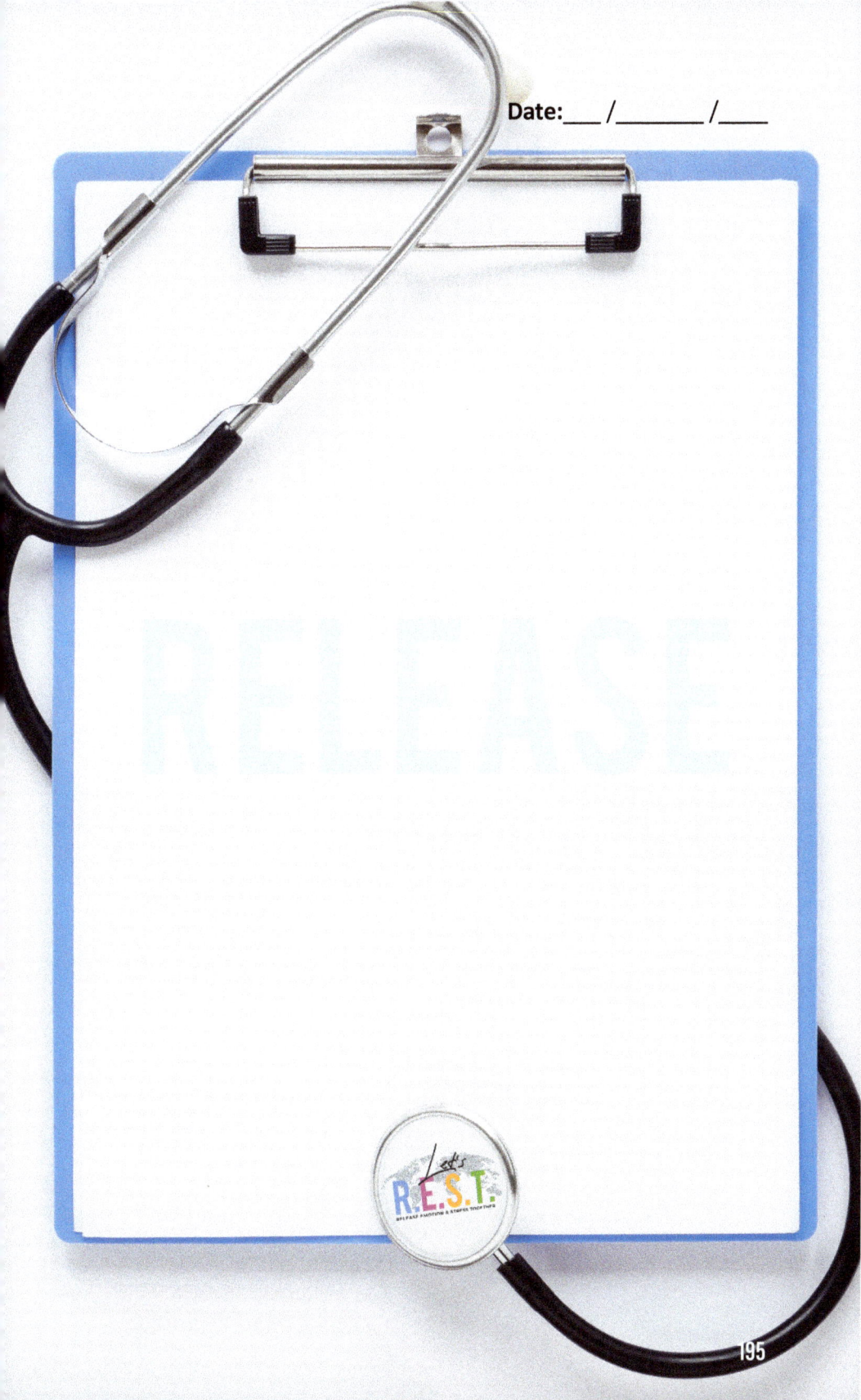

Date:___ /_____ /___

RELEASE

In order to seize our tomorrow, I believe that we must prepare today.
In preparation for tomorrow, I've discovered
that our todays give many lessons.
When we embrace the lessons of today, we are strengthened
emotionally and physically for our tomorrow.
Therefore, the victory for tomorrow is in the submitting to the
inner change and transformation from the lessons of our today.

— —Dr. Chevelta A. Smith

What did you learn **TODAY**, and *how* will you apply this knowledge to become a better/healthier you **TOMORROW?**

Let's R.E.S.T. **Bedtime Affirmation**
(Say it out loud!)

I am strong!
I am resilient!
I am able to overcome every disappointment and setback from today
I am more than a conqueror!
I will recharge myself with good sleep tonight
I will awake with a renewed sense of purpose
And I declare that my tomorrow will be great!

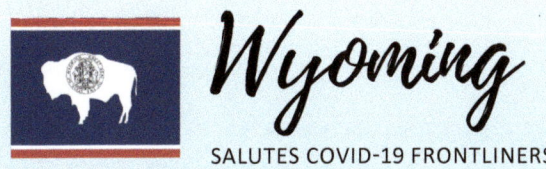

Wyoming
SALUTES COVID-19 FRONTLINERS

Several years ago, while visiting my grandparents' graves, I chose to idly wander among nearby graves. By chance, I came upon a family plot where a father, mother, and son were laid to rest. The father and son died within a month of each other while the mother did not pass until some thirty years later. Both the father and son were physicians that died during the 1918 Influenza Pandemic with the father in his fifties and the son his twenties. I remember pondering what courage and compassion must have existed within those souls. I believe I now better understand. I saw that same courage and compassion with our medical providers facing down the terror of COVID-19. This generation, as well as future generations, will recognize your courageous and compassionate achievements. We are so forever grateful. Thank you!"

—Anonymous
Cheyenne, Wyoming

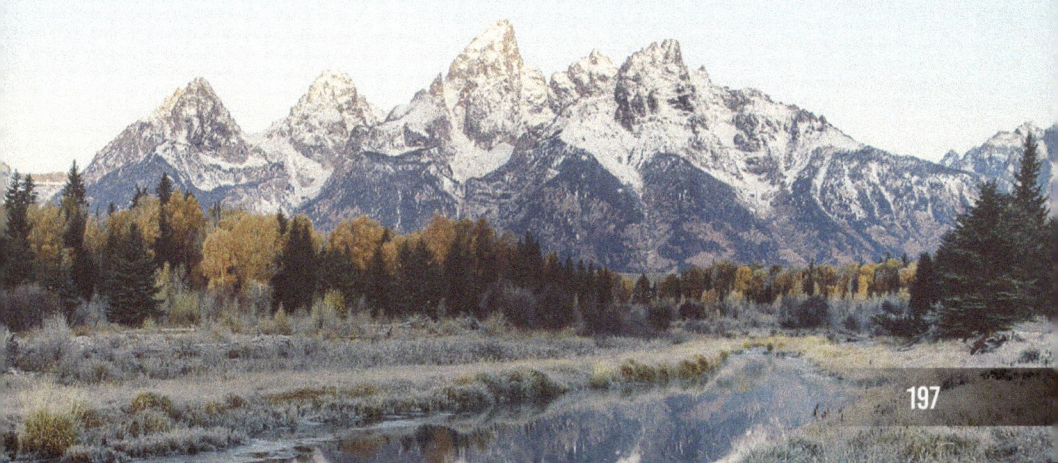

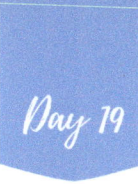

Day 19

MORNING HUDDLE

When You Strengthen Your Mental Immunity…You Will Resist Every Hindrance, Distraction, and Trap That Is Meant to Hold You Back.

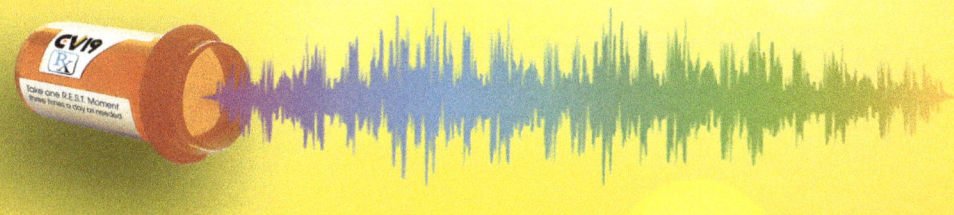

"It's all about your mindset and developing one that is strong!"

—Dr. Chevelta A. Smith

7:38 Min

MENTAL IMMUNITY

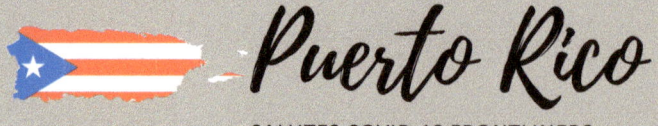

Puerto Rico
SALUTES COVID-19 FRONTLINERS

"Hemos sido puestos a prueba este año. No importa de donde venimos o donde vivimos, todos estamos en esta lucha juntos. Para los que estamos tratando de volver a la normalidad, les recuerdo que somos más fuertes si permanecemos unidos y pensando de manera positiva. Pensemos en un mejor futuro y en un mundo donde todos nos valoremos y amamemos los unos a los otros".

English version:

We have been greatly tested this year. No matter where we come from or live, we are all in this fight together. For those of us working to return to a sense of normalcy, I remind you that we are stronger united and with a positive mindset. Let us look forward to a better future and a world where we all appreciate and love each other.

—Ruth T.
Ponce, Puerto Rico

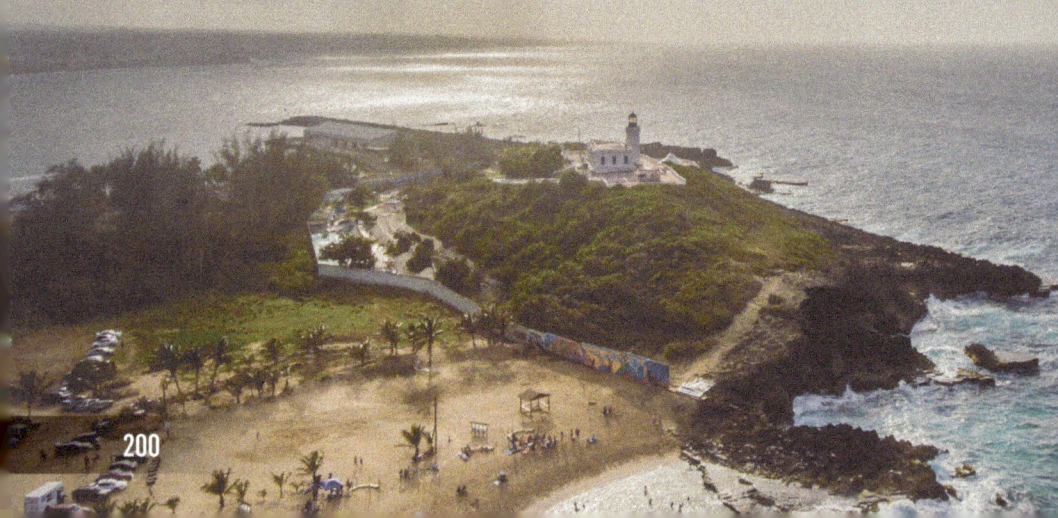

R — Today I RELEASED my... *(check all that apply)*

Mind By:
- Communicating my thoughts, feelings, & needs to others
- Speaking positive self-affirmations
- Deep breathing
- Other _____

Body By:
- Muscle Relaxation Techniques
- Exercise
- Hydrotherapy: bath or shower
- Other _____

Spirit By:
- Meditation
- Journaling
- Praying
- Going outside for 15-20 minutes
- Self-Talk
- Other _____

E — Today I FEEL... *(circle one)*

Happy / Anger / Love / Sad / Fear

Surprise / Disgust / Trust / Anticipation

Other _____

What is your dominant **EMOTION** in your life right now?

S

What were your main **STRESSORS** today?

What *Methods* are you using today **TO REDUCE** your current stress?

What *Value* have you noticed **IN USING** them?

T — Stick TOGETHER: How did you *Connect* today?

- Reached out to a co-worker who appeared to be struggling
- Expressed openly with trusted family or co-workers about how the pandemic is affecting me
- Identified factors that are overwhelming/stressful and worked with others to find solutions
- Initiated the "Buddy" System with other co-workers and monitored each other for signs of stress, burnout, and depression
- Spoke to a mental health care provider

My *Let's* **R.E.S.T.** *Affirmation for Today:*

My mind is strong! I am emotionally resilient. I can do anything I put my mind to.

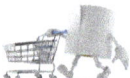 What do you need, but feel like it's unavailable?

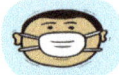 What are you having a hard time expressing?

 Who or what have you distanced yourself from that could help you overcome the above struggles/difficulties?

 **NEXT STEPS: Make a healthy plan of action that you will implement in order to help protect yourself from being overtaken by the daily stress of the pandemic.** _____
_____
_____
_____
_____
_____
_____

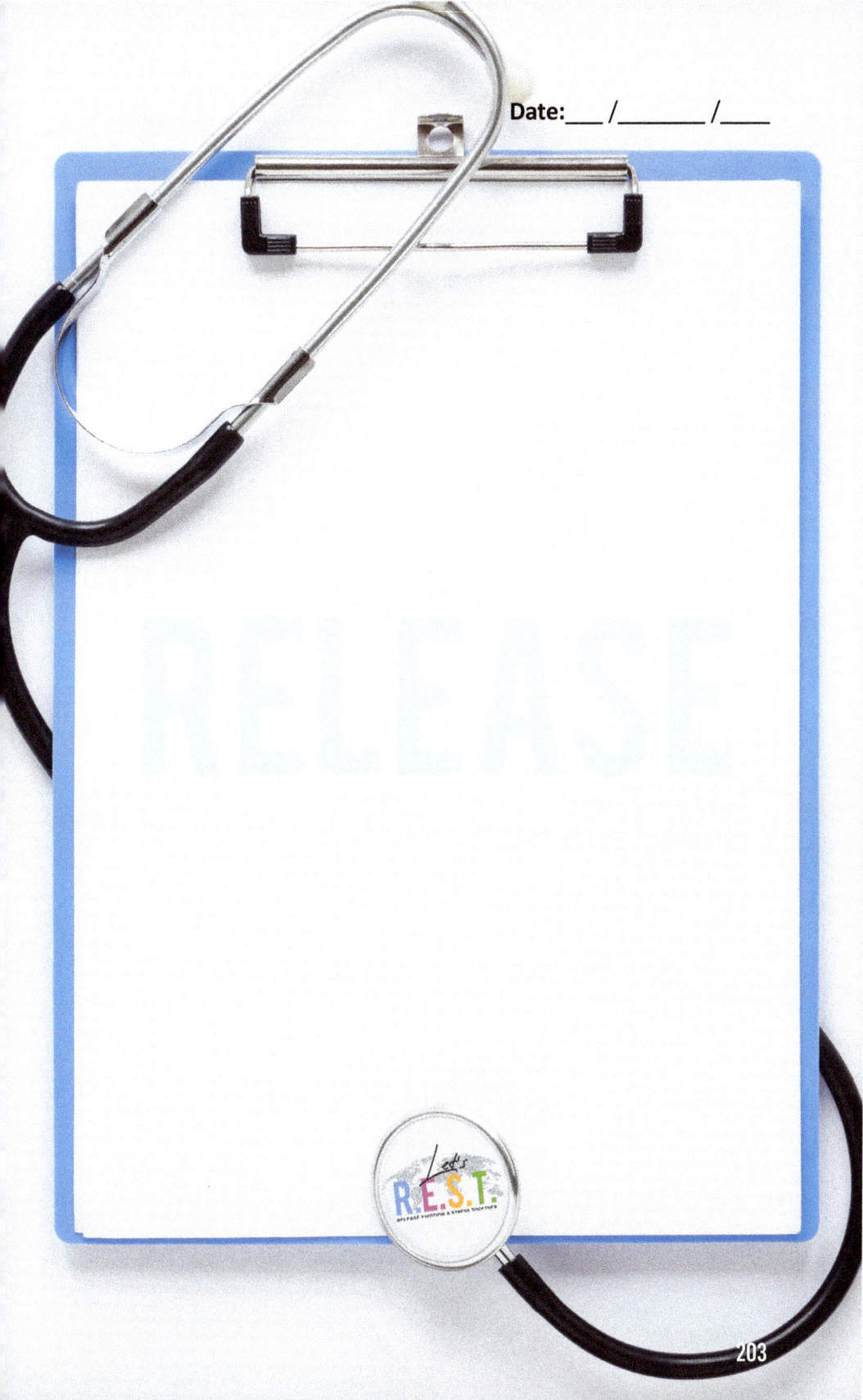

Date:___ / _____ / ___

RELEASE

In order to seize our tomorrow, I believe that we must prepare today.
In preparation for tomorrow, I've discovered
that our todays give many lessons.
When we embrace the lessons of today, we are strengthened
emotionally and physically for our tomorrow.
Therefore, the victory for tomorrow is in the submitting to the
inner change and transformation from the lessons of our today.

—— Dr. Chevelta A. Smith

What did you learn **TODAY,** and *how* will you apply this knowledge to become a better/healthier you **TOMORROW?**

Let's R.E.S.T. **Bedtime Affirmation**
(Say it out loud!)

I am strong!
I am resilient!
I am able to overcome every disappointment and setback from today
I am more than a conqueror!
I will recharge myself with good sleep tonight
I will awake with a renewed sense of purpose
And I declare that my tomorrow will be great!

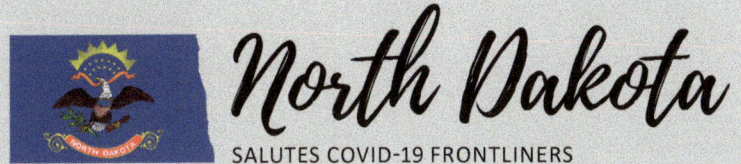

North Dakota

SALUTES COVID-19 FRONTLINERS

Dear First Responder,

First, I want to say thank you. Thank you for your bravery. I'm sure that when you took your oath, you knew that came with some risk and that you could possibly risk your life while trying to help save the lives of others. However, I am also almost certain that you had no idea that it would come to this: That every day you would be faced with an overwhelming amount of death due to COVID-19 (let alone put your life and immediate family's life at risk due to this silent killer). Yet, every day you [warrior] go on to do the work you were called to do. I know your work has taken a toll on you physically due to the long hours and limited downtime between patients due to this virus. I cannot begin to imagine the toll it has taken on your mind.

Please take comfort in knowing that I am sincerely praying for your physical and emotional wellbeing. I cannot say thank you enough for doing the work that many of us aren't able to or are too afraid to do. Thank you. May God keep you and bring you out stronger on the other side of this.
Sincerely,

—Chante C.
Minor, North Dakota

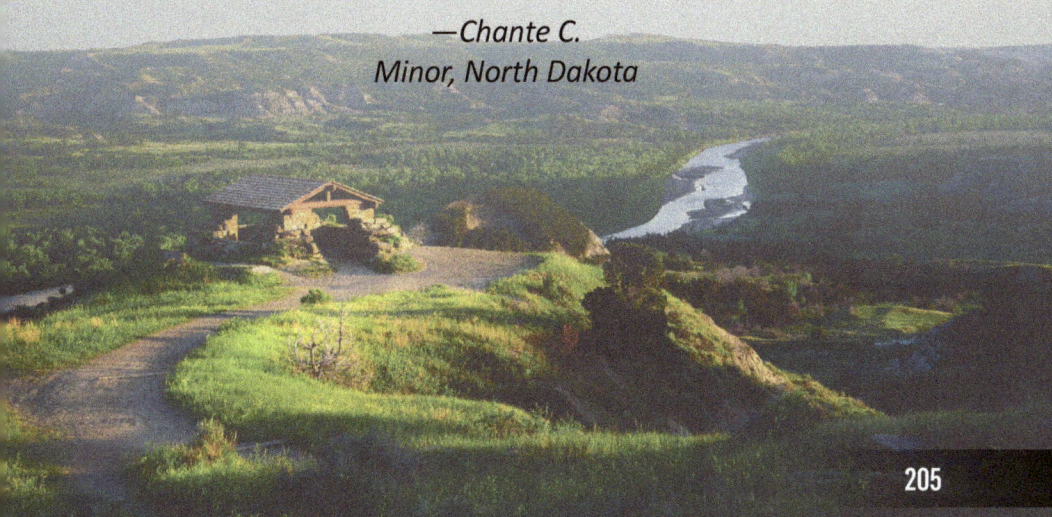

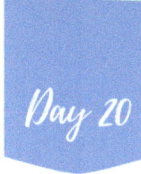

Day 20

MORNING HUDDLE

Some Things Happened Yesterday That You Are Still Holding Onto Today. Release Yesterday.

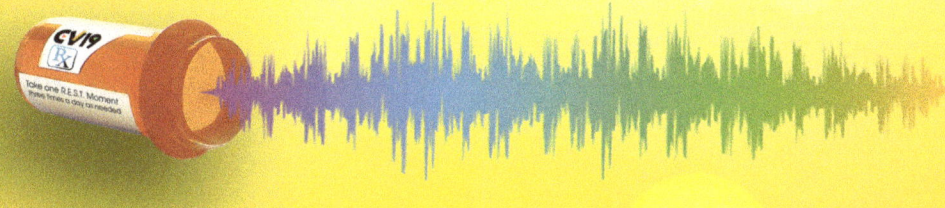

"Release yourself from the things that are hindering your ability to love yourself and embrace who you are in the fullest."
—Dr. Chevelta A. Smith

AFFIRMATION RELEASE

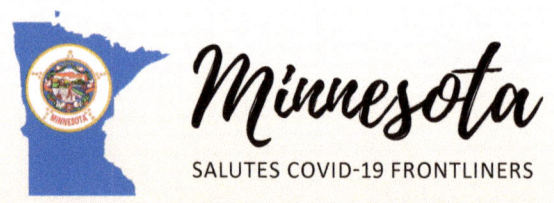

Minnesota
SALUTES COVID-19 FRONTLINERS

May you be strengthened daily; your fears calmed; and your spirits lifted, in knowing, that you are angels of mercy to those who are sick.

May you realize and see the light at the end of the tunnel. Every storm has its ending, this one will too.

May God bless you and keep you healthy.

—Anonymous.
Cokato, Minnesota

R — Today I RELEASED my... (check all that apply)

Mind By:
- Communicating my thoughts, feelings, & needs to others
- Speaking positive self-affirmations
- Deep breathing
- Other _____

Body By:
- Muscle Relaxation Techniques
- Exercise
- Hydrotherapy: bath or shower
- Other _____

Spirit By:
- Meditation
- Journaling
- Praying
- Going outside for 15-20 minutes
- Self-Talk
- Other _____

E — Today I FEEL... (circle one)

Happy / Anger / Love / Sad / Fear

Surprise / Disgust / Trust / Anticipation

Other _____

What is your dominant **EMOTION** in your life right now?

S

What were your main **STRESSORS** today?

What *Methods* are you using today **TO REDUCE** your current stress?

What *Value* have you noticed **IN USING** them?

T — Stick TOGETHER: How did you *Connect* today?

- Reached out to a co-worker who appeared to be struggling
- Expressed openly with trusted family or co-workers about how the pandemic is affecting me
- Identified factors that are overwhelming/stressful and worked with others to find solutions
- Initiated the "Buddy" System with other co-workers and monitored each other for signs of stress, burnout, and depression
- Spoke to a mental health care provider

My *Let's* R.E.S.T. Affirmation for Today:

I release myself from the fear of failure and self-doubt! I release anxiety, worry, and stress.

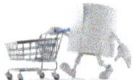 What do you need, but feel like it's unavailable?

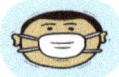 What are you having a hard time expressing?

 Who or what have you distanced yourself from that could help you overcome the above struggles/difficulties?

 **NEXT STEPS: Make a healthy plan of action that you will implement in order to help protect yourself from being overtaken by the daily stress of the pandemic.** _____
_____
_____
_____
_____
_____

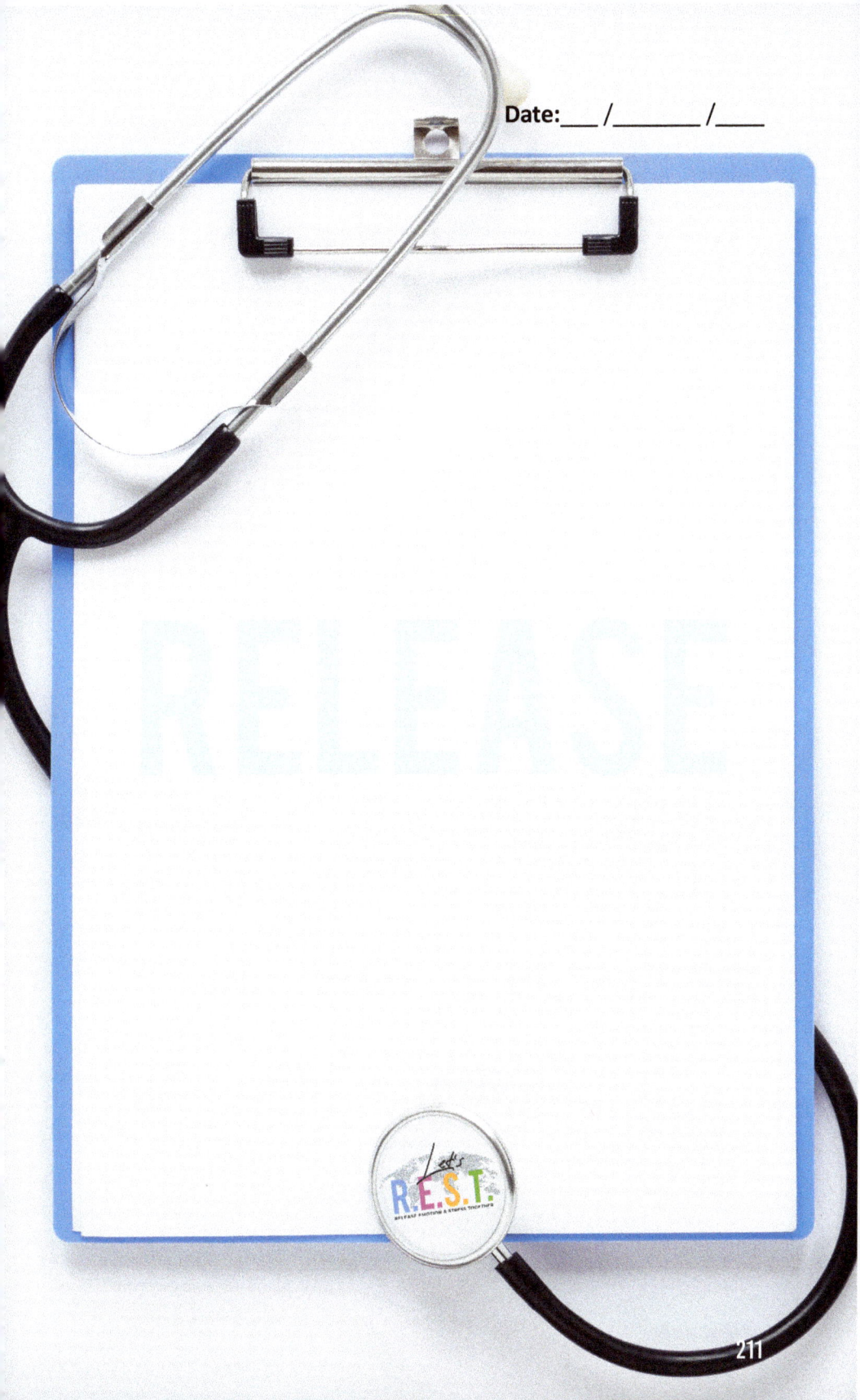

In order to seize our tomorrow, I believe that we must prepare today.
In preparation for tomorrow, I've discovered
that our todays give many lessons.
When we embrace the lessons of today, we are strengthened
emotionally and physically for our tomorrow.
Therefore, the victory for tomorrow is in the submitting to the
inner change and transformation from the lessons of our today.

--Dr. Chevelta A. Smith

What did you learn **TODAY**, and *how* will you apply this knowledge to become a better/healthier you **TOMORROW?**

Let's R.E.S.T. **Bedtime Affirmation**
(Say it out loud!)

I am strong!
I am resilient!
I am able to overcome every disappointment and setback from today
I am more than a conqueror!
I will recharge myself with good sleep tonight
I will awake with a renewed sense of purpose
And I declare that my tomorrow will be great!

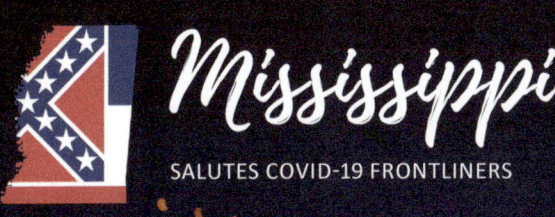

Mississippi
SALUTES COVID-19 FRONTLINERS

God uses special people in special places to help others in need, so thank you for accepting your special assignment on the frontlines. My prayer is that God will bless all of the frontline workers!

—Dr. Denecise S.
Tupelo, Mississippi

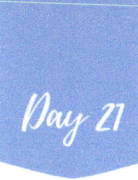

Day 21

MORNING HUDDLE

If You Don't Slow Down and Take Time for Yourself, Then it May Not Matter That You're Born to Do Something Great Because Your Body May Give Out on You, Making You Unable to Complete Your Purpose on This Earth.

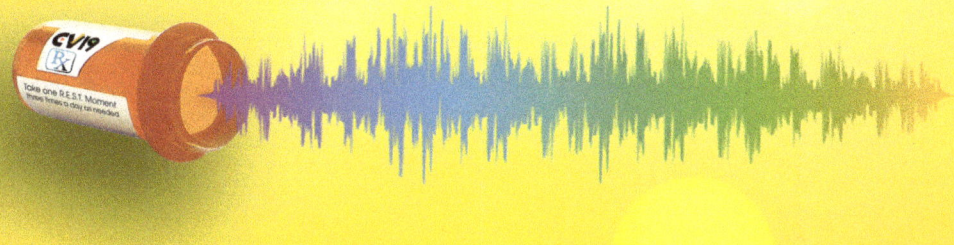

"Maybe it's a good thing that I don't know what to do!"
—Dr. Chevelta A. Smith

SLOW DOWN

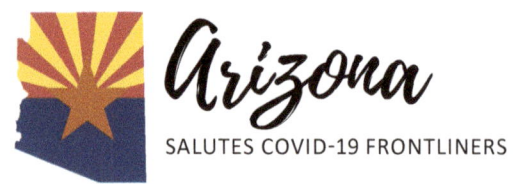

Arizona
SALUTES COVID-19 FRONTLINERS

Thank you for ALL of the sacrifices you make daily! You all are extremely special people who are the first to selflessly respond to our pains & illnesses. We pray that you all will soon be refreshed, and your strength quickly replenished sooner than later. Additionally, for the other unsung heroes and heroines whose jobs support the medical professionals, you too are appreciated, loved, and cherished. God's blessings belong to each of you. Psalms 91

—Vanessa S.
Phoenix, Arizona

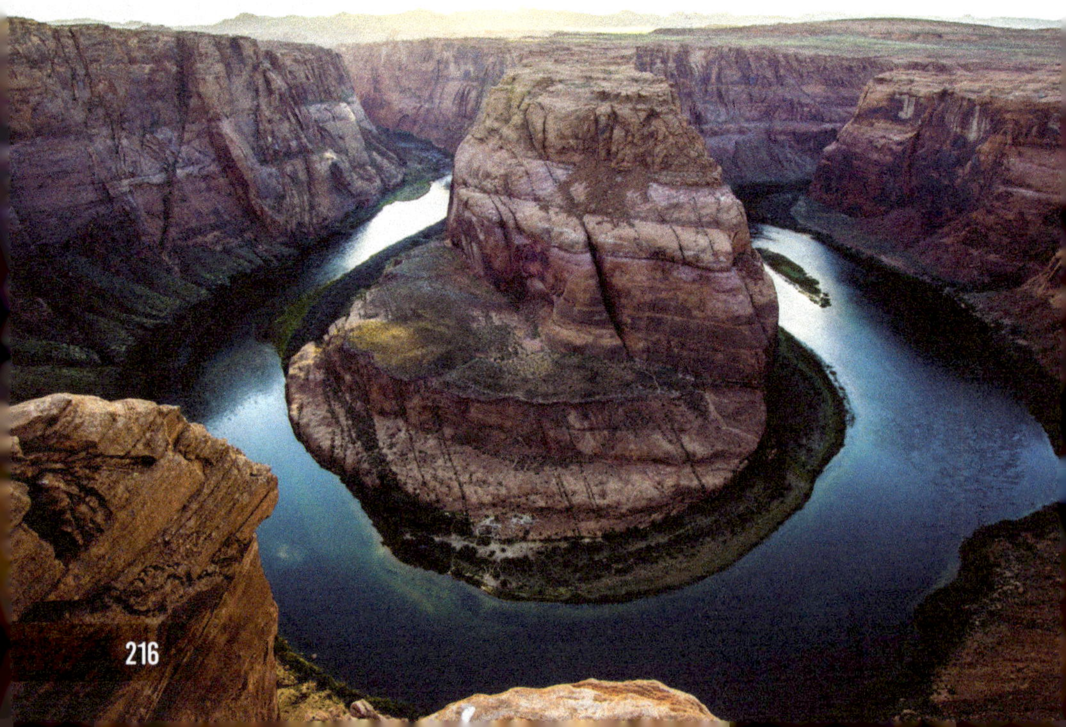

R — Today I RELEASED my... (check all that apply)

Mind By:
- ■ Communicating my thoughts, feelings, & needs to others
- ■ Speaking positive self-affirmations ■ Deep breathing ■ Other _____

Body By:
- ■ Muscle Relaxation Techniques ■ Exercise
- ■ Hydrotherapy: bath or shower ■ Other _____

Spirit By:
- ■ Meditation ■ Journaling ■ Praying
- ■ Going outside for 15-20 minutes ■ Self-Talk ■ Other _____

E — Today I FEEL... (circle one)

Happy / Anger / Love / Sad / Fear

Surprise / Disgust / Trust / Anticipation

Other _____

What is your dominant **EMOTION** in your life right now?

S

What were your main **STRESSORS** today?

What *Methods* are you using today **TO REDUCE** your current stress?

What *Value* have you noticed **IN USING** them?

T — Stick TOGETHER: How did you *Connect* today?

- ○ Reached out to a co-worker who appeared to be struggling
- ○ Expressed openly with trusted family or co-workers about how the pandemic is affecting me
- ○ Identified factors that are overwhelming/stressful and worked with others to find solutions
- ○ Initiated the "Buddy" System with other co-workers and monitored each other for signs of stress, burnout, and depression
- ○ Spoke to a mental health care provider

My *Let's* R.E.S.T. Affirmation for Today:

Today, I will be good to myself. I will take a moment to slow down and refuel my body, soul, and spirit

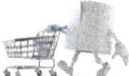 What do you need, but feel like it's unavailable?

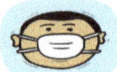 What are you having a hard time expressing?

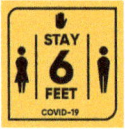 Who or what have you distanced yourself from that could help you overcome the above struggles/difficulties?

 NEXT STEPS: Make a healthy plan of action that you will implement in order to help protect yourself from being overtaken by the daily stress of the pandemic. _____
_____
_____
_____
_____
_____

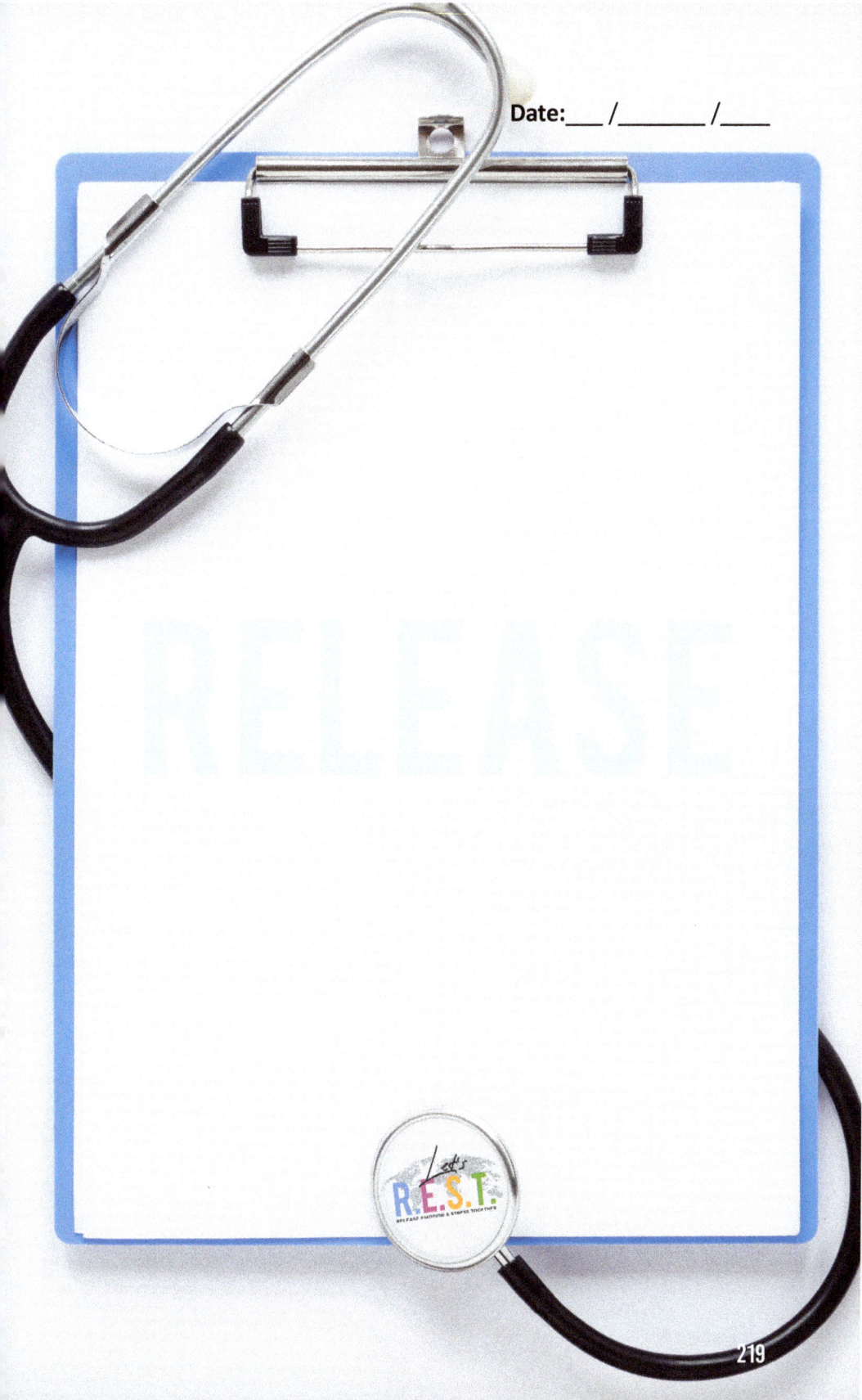

Date:___ / _____ / ___

In order to seize our tomorrow, I believe that we must prepare today.
In preparation for tomorrow, I've discovered
that our todays give many lessons.
When we embrace the lessons of today, we are strengthened
emotionally and physically for our tomorrow.
Therefore, the victory for tomorrow is in the submitting to the
inner change and transformation from the lessons of our today.

--Dr. Chevelta A. Smith

What did you learn **TODAY**, and *how* will you apply this knowledge to become a better/healthier you **TOMORROW?**

Let's R.E.S.T. **Bedtime Affirmation**
(Say it out loud!)

I am strong!
I am resilient!
I am able to overcome every disappointment and setback from today
I am more than a conqueror!
I will recharge myself with good sleep tonight
I will awake with a renewed sense of purpose
And I declare that my tomorrow will be great!

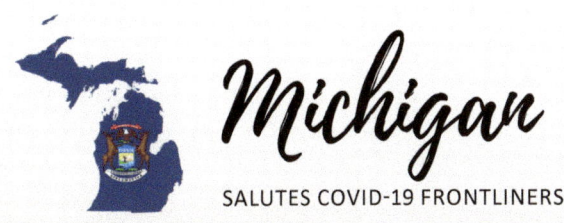

Michigan
SALUTES COVID-19 FRONTLINERS

The term "essential" has taken on a metamorphosis in the last 5 months. Prior to the global, Novel Corona-19 pandemic, the use of this term generally described something to be placed in a priority status on a "to do list." Your passionate, purposeful, selfless, and sacrificial use of your invaluable skills to maintain and preserve life has eclipsed our prior understanding of the term essential and its meaning. You now provoke sentiments parallel to the sanctity of life itself. Your essentialism is the essence of life for many.

—*Nicolas S.*
Detroit, Michigan

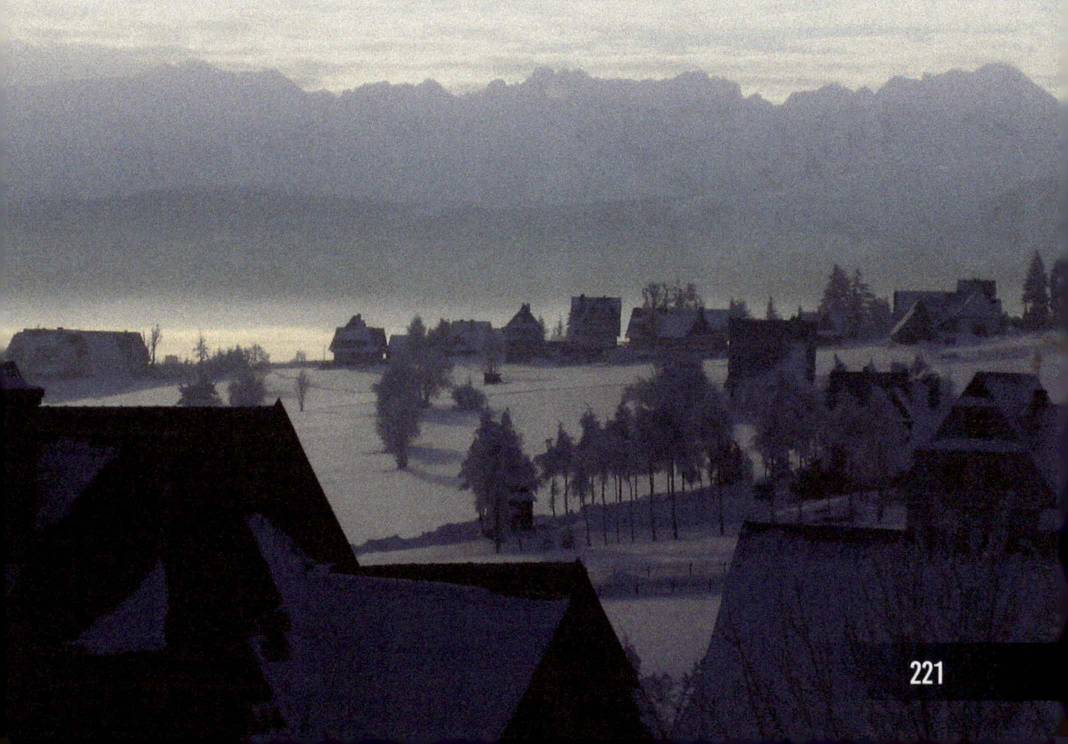

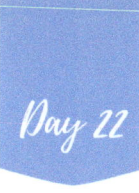

Day 22

MORNING HUDDLE

Take Time to Rest Physically.
Take Time to Rest Mentally.
Take Time to Rest Spiritually.

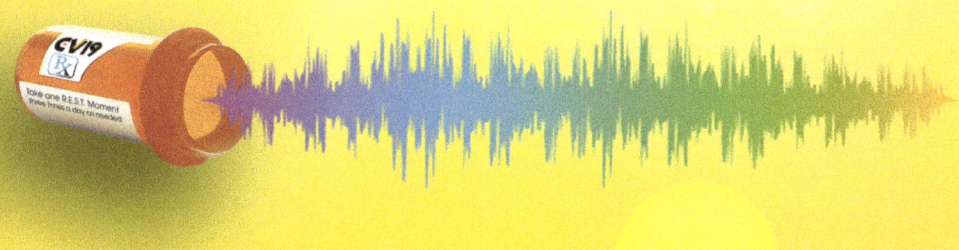

"Be careful that you don't internalize your stress, your feelings, or your worries."

—Dr. Chevelta A. Smith

REST

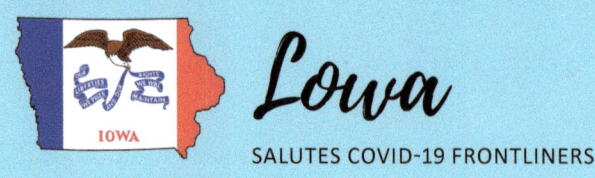

Iowa

SALUTES COVID-19 FRONTLINERS

Thank you for your hard work and dedication through the COVID-19 pandemic. Putting your health at risk is something you're familiar with but, probably not to this scale. I don't only mean the concern of being infected by the virus, but the stress of the unknown and juggling new and changing procedures and environments on a near-daily basis. I applaud you for the work you're doing. Rest when you can, I know you're tired, take care of yourself, because the ones you care for need you to stay mentally and emotionally happy as well at work and at home.

—Amber K.
Mount Pleasant, Iowa

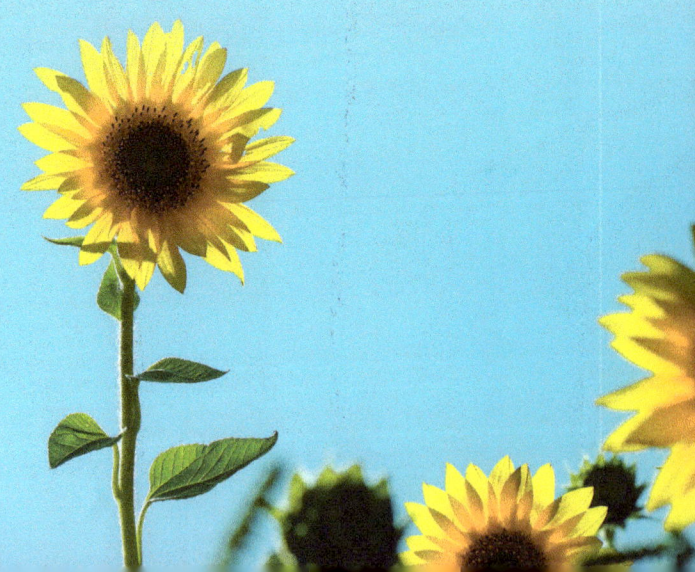

R

Today **I RELEASED** *my*... *(check all that apply)*

Mind By:
- ■ Communicating my thoughts, feelings, & needs to others
- ■ Speaking positive self-affirmations ■ Deep breathing ■ Other _____

Body By:
- ■ Muscle Relaxation Techniques ■ Exercise
- ■ Hydrotherapy: bath or shower ■ Other _____

Spirit By:
- ■ Meditation ■ Journaling ■ Praying
- ■ Going outside for 15-20 minutes ■ Self-Talk ■ Other _____

E

Today **I FEEL**... *(circle one)*

Happy / Anger / Love / Sad / Fear

Surprise / Disgust / Trust / Anticipation

Other _____

What is your dominant **EMOTION** in your life right now?

S

What were your main **STRESSORS** today?

What *Methods* are you using today **TO REDUCE** your current stress?

What *Value* have you noticed **IN USING** them?

T

Stick TOGETHER: How did you *Connect* today?

- ○ Reached out to a co-worker who appeared to be struggling
- ○ Expressed openly with trusted family or co-workers about how the pandemic is affecting me
- ○ Identified factors that are overwhelming/stressful and worked with others to find solutions
- ○ Initiated the "Buddy" System with other co-workers and monitored each other for signs of stress, burnout, and depression
- ○ Spoke to a mental health care provider

My *Let's* **R.E.S.T.** *Affirmation for Today:*

I will quiet my mind from the stress and anxiety of today. I will relax and recharge. I will have peaceful sleep tonight.

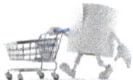 What do you need, but feel like it's unavailable?

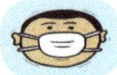 What are you having a hard time expressing?

 Who or what have you distanced yourself from that could help you overcome the above struggles/difficulties?

 NEXT STEPS: Make a healthy plan of action that you will implement in order to help protect yourself from being overtaken by the daily stress of the pandemic. _____
_____
_____
_____
_____
_____

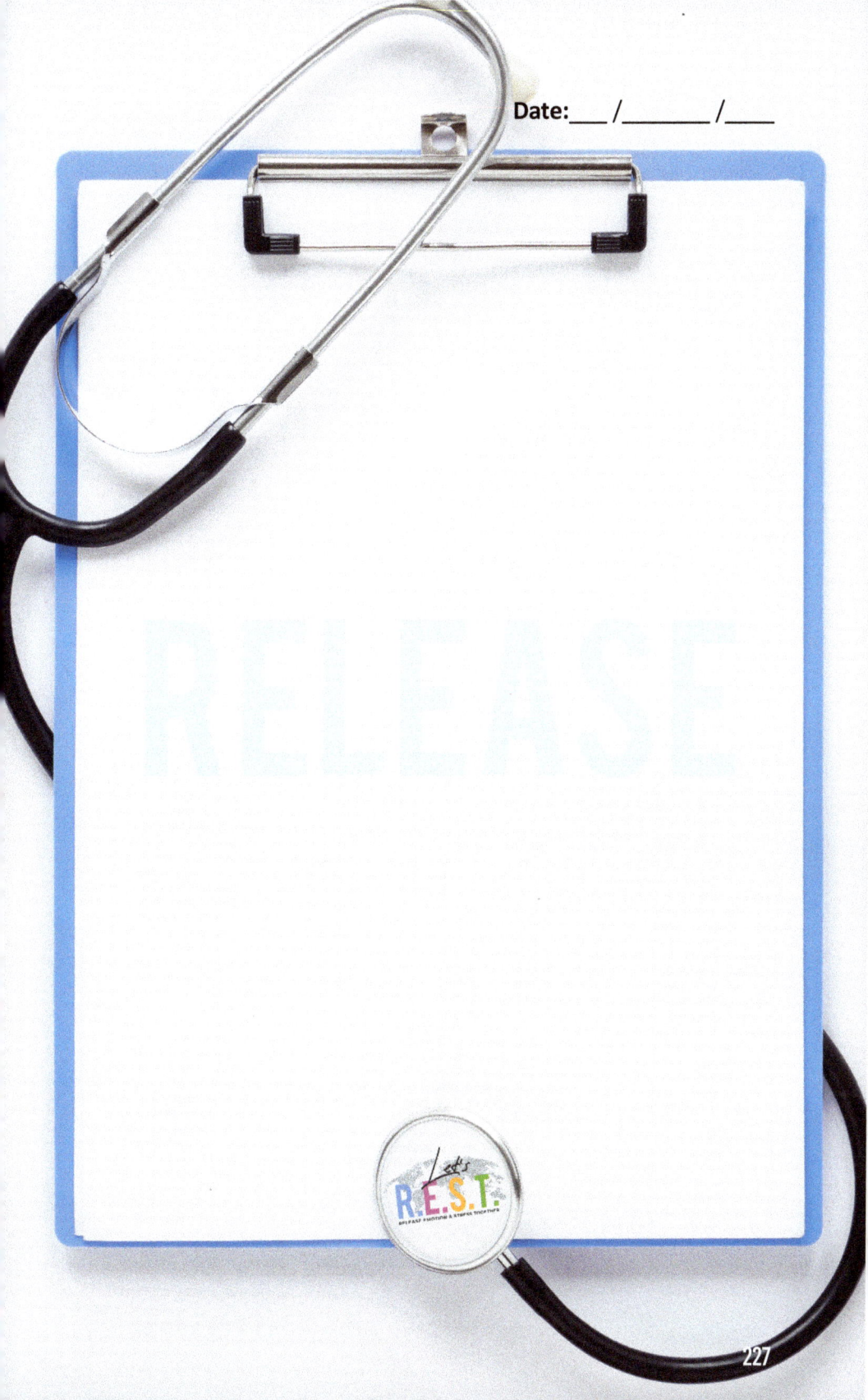

Date:___ /_____ /____

In order to seize our tomorrow, I believe that we must prepare today.
In preparation for tomorrow, I've discovered
that our todays give many lessons.
When we embrace the lessons of today, we are strengthened
emotionally and physically for our tomorrow.
Therefore, the victory for tomorrow is in the submitting to the
inner change and transformation from the lessons of our today.

— Dr. Chevelta A. Smith

What did you learn **TODAY**, and *how* will you apply this knowledge to become a better/healthier you **TOMORROW?**

Let's R.E.S.T. **Bedtime Affirmation**
(Say it out loud!)

I am strong!
I am resilient!
I am able to overcome every disappointment and setback from today
I am more than a conqueror!
I will recharge myself with good sleep tonight
I will awake with a renewed sense of purpose
And I declare that my tomorrow will be great!

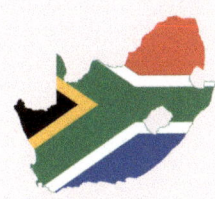 SALUTES COVID-19 FRONTLINERS

I would like to encourage the Medical Frontliners to keep up the good work. They keep showing up regardless of the outcomes and that is something that a lot of people struggle to do for their own lives; but the frontliners do it restlessly to save the lives of others. They need to know that with God everything is possible. The storm will always pass as it always has. Pandemics have come and gone so they need not underestimate the value of their efforts with the current one.

Medical professionals are the solution to every one of our medical crises and will always be. There is a reason God allowed the medical profession to manifest, and in my opinion it is because it is crucial to our existence.

Take Care and God Bless,
—Venus
South Africa

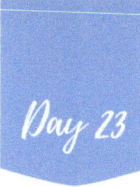

Day 23

MORNING HUDDLE

Release Fear. Release Unforgiveness. Release Yourself to Be Free. Hold Onto Love. Hold Onto Strength. Hold Onto Everything and Everyone That Makes You Become All That You Are Suppose to Be

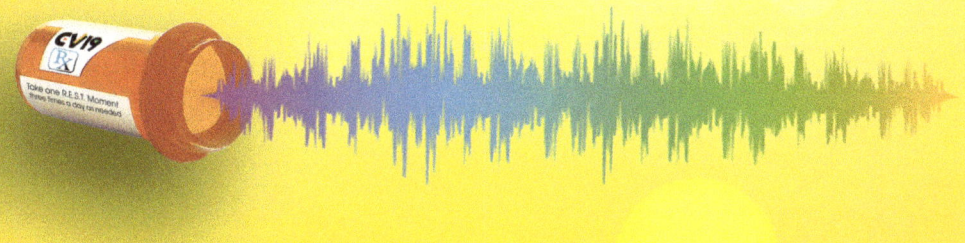

"You have the power and the freedom to choose what thoughts you will buy into."

—Dr. Chevelta A. Smith

HOLD & RELEASE

Delaware
SALUTES COVID-19 FRONTLINERS

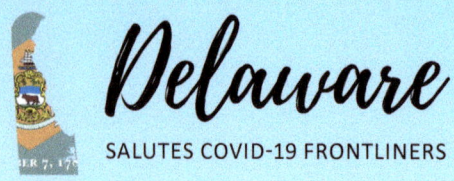

*I just want to say to all the frontline hospital workers, even down to the janitors, hold on!!
Keep the faith! We appreciate you.
We are praying daily for you all. I love you. Strength to you all.*

—Darlene S.
Dover, Delaware

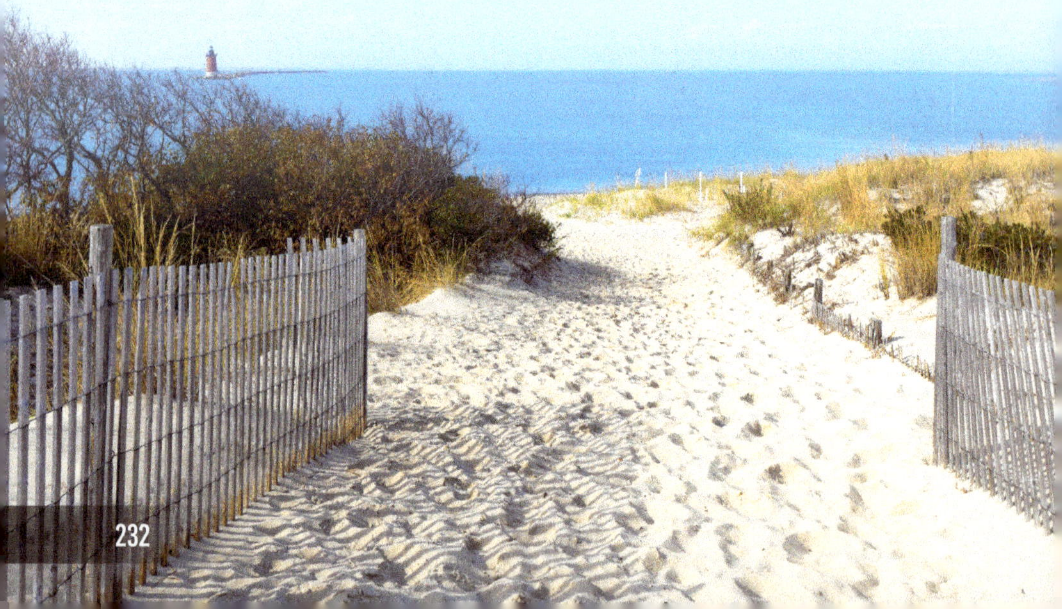

R — Today I RELEASED my... (check all that apply)

Mind By:
- ☐ Communicating my thoughts, feelings, & needs to others
- ☐ Speaking positive self-affirmations ☐ Deep breathing ☐ Other _____

Body By:
- ☐ Muscle Relaxation Techniques ☐ Exercise
- ☐ Hydrotherapy: bath or shower ☐ Other _____

Spirit By:
- ☐ Meditation ☐ Journaling ☐ Praying
- ☐ Going outside for 15-20 minutes ☐ Self-Talk ☐ Other _____

E — Today I FEEL... (circle one)

Happy / Anger / Love / Sad / Fear

Surprise / Disgust / Trust / Anticipation

Other _____

What is your dominant EMOTION in your life right now?

S

What were your main STRESSORS today?

What *Methods* are you using today TO REDUCE your current stress?

What *Value* have you noticed IN USING them?

T — Stick TOGETHER: How did you *Connect* today?

- ○ Reached out to a co-worker who appeared to be struggling
- ○ Expressed openly with trusted family or co-workers about how the pandemic is affecting me
- ○ Identified factors that are overwhelming/stressful and worked with others to find solutions
- ○ Initiated the "Buddy" System with other co-workers and monitored each other for signs of stress, burnout, and depression
- ○ Spoke to a mental health care provider

My *Let's* R.E.S.T. *Affirmation for Today:*
I will hold on to strength, peace, and compassion. I release fear and stress.

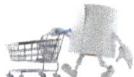 What do you need, but feel like it's unavailable?

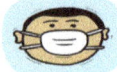 What are you having a hard time expressing?

 Who or what have you distanced yourself from that could help you overcome the above struggles/difficulties?

 **NEXT STEPS: Make a healthy plan of action that you will implement in order to help protect yourself from being overtaken by the daily stress of the pandemic.** _____
_____
_____
_____
_____
_____
_____

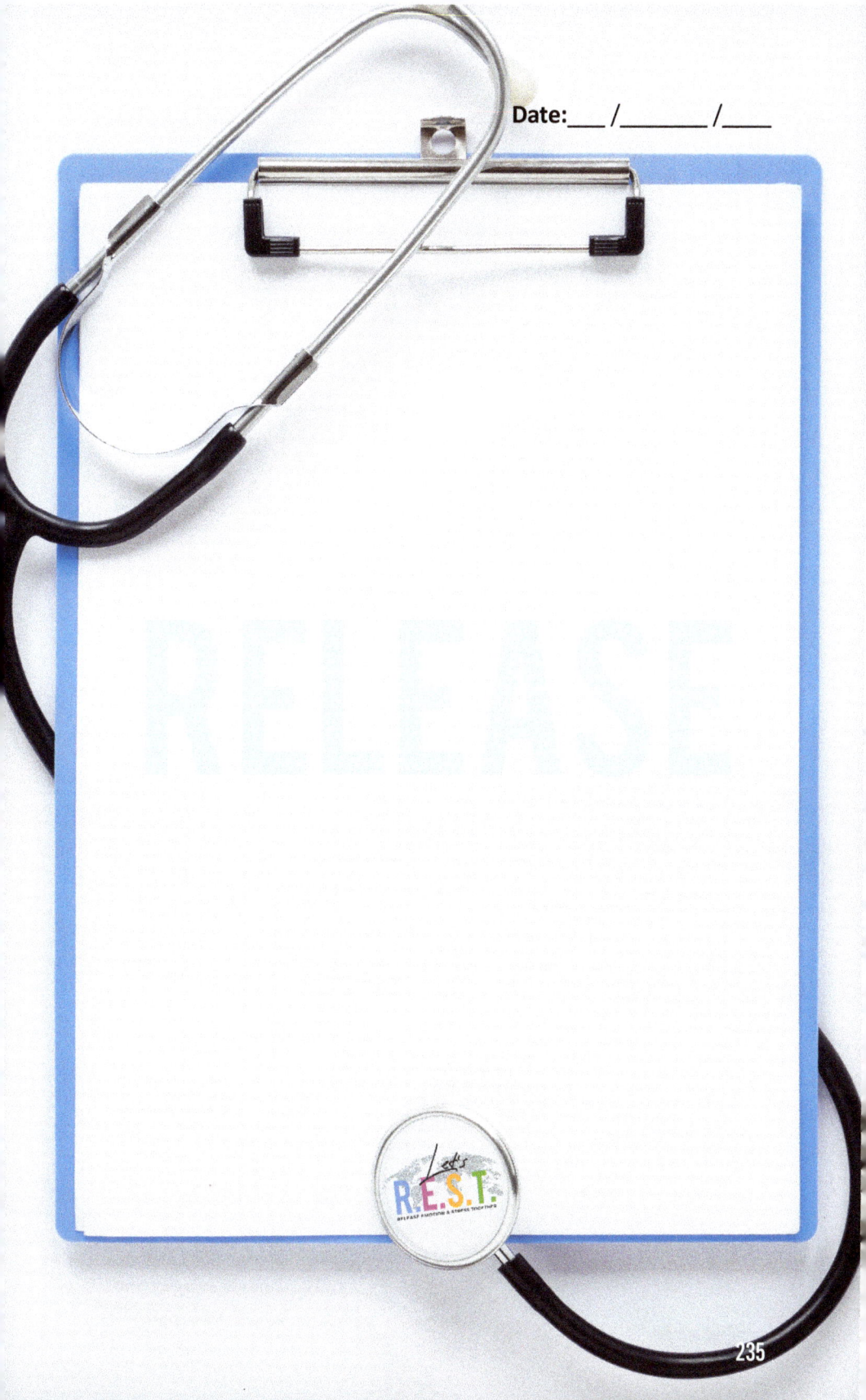

In order to seize our tomorrow, I believe that we must prepare today.
In preparation for tomorrow, I've discovered
that our todays give many lessons.
When we embrace the lessons of today, we are strengthened
emotionally and physically for our tomorrow.
Therefore, the victory for tomorrow is in the submitting to the
inner change and transformation from the lessons of our today.

--Dr. Chevelta A. Smith

What did you learn **TODAY,** and *how* will you apply this knowledge to become a better/healthier you **TOMORROW?**

Let's R.E.S.T. **Bedtime Affirmation**
(Say it out loud!)

I am strong!
I am resilient!
I am able to overcome every disappointment and setback from today
I am more than a conqueror!
I will recharge myself with good sleep tonight
I will awake with a renewed sense of purpose
And I declare that my tomorrow will be great!

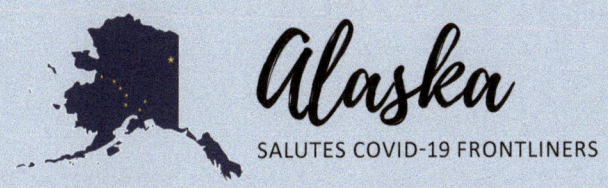

Alaska
SALUTES COVID-19 FRONTLINERS

Dear Frontliners!!!!!

I remember watching YouTube videos from China when the virus was first discovered back in January. How blessed I felt knowing we were in the US. I can't express the gratitude I have towards all the medical professionals who continually return to their place of employment fighting this aggressive virus. To be surrounded by the smell of death and increasing your chances of contracting it, not many would be willing to continue to do.

You are more than essential, and we are so blessed to live here in America and have access to willing and compassionate medical professionals!

Prayers for all of you from Palmer, Alaska
—Kelly G.

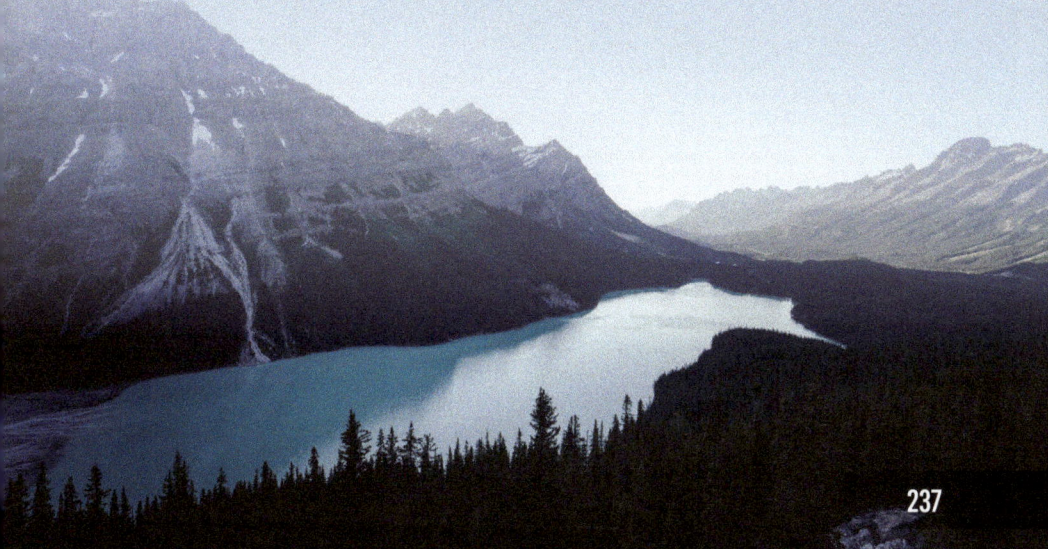

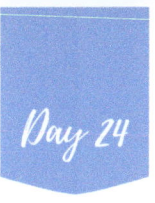

Day 24

MORNING HUDDLE

Strength. It's What Allows You to Move Forth in Courage.
Courage. The Action Every Frontliner Takes to Save Lives.

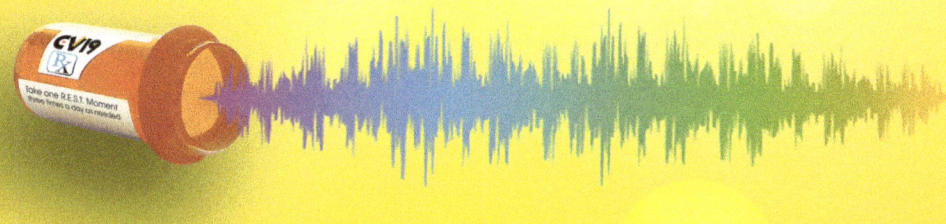

"That courage looks good on you!"
—Dr. Chevelta A. Smith

AFFIRMATION COURAGE

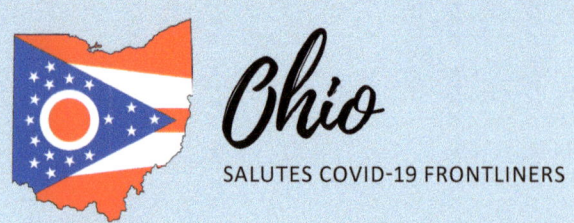

Ohio
SALUTES COVID-19 FRONTLINERS

To everyone fighting the battle against COVID-19,

Thank you so much for doing God's work. I pray that you'll receive His protection as you stand on the frontlines in the battle against this illness.

There's a quote that "Courage is not the absence of fear, but rather the judgment that something else is more important than one's fear." You are certainly courageous, and our country owes you their eternal gratitude.
Keep fighting the good fight!

Somewhere outside Cincinnati, Ohio.
—Jamie J.

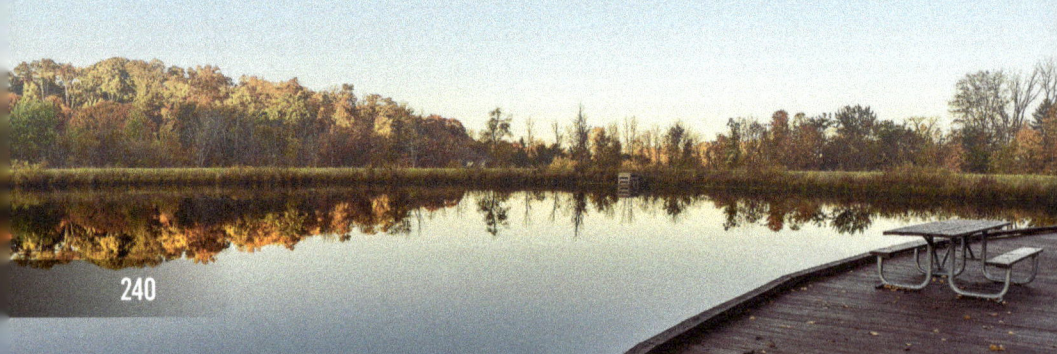

R

Today I RELEASED my... (check all that apply)

Mind By:
- ■ Communicating my thoughts, feelings, & needs to others
- ■ Speaking positive self-affirmations ■ Deep breathing ■ Other _____

Body By:
- ■ Muscle Relaxation Techniques   ■ Exercise
- ■ Hydrotherapy: bath or shower   ■ Other _____

Spirit By:
- ■ Meditation   ■ Journaling   ■ Praying
- ■ Going outside for 15-20 minutes   ■ Self-Talk   ■ Other _____

E

Today I FEEL... (circle one)

Happy / Anger / Love / Sad / Fear

Surprise / Disgust / Trust / Anticipation

Other _____

What is your dominant **EMOTION** in your life right now?

S

What were your main **STRESSORS** today?

What *Methods* are you using today **TO REDUCE** your current stress?

What *Value* have you noticed **IN USING** them?

T

Stick TOGETHER: How did you *Connect* today?

- ○ Reached out to a co-worker who appeared to be struggling
- ○ Expressed openly with trusted family or co-workers about how the pandemic is affecting me
- ○ Identified factors that are overwhelming/stressful and worked with others to find solutions
- ○ Initiated the "Buddy" System with other co-workers and monitored each other for signs of stress, burnout, and depression
- ○ Spoke to a mental health care provider

My *Let's* R.E.S.T. Affirmation for Today:

I am brave and fearless. I am making an amazing difference in the lives of others, through my courage.

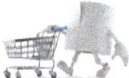
What do you need, but feel like it's unavailable?

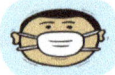
What are you having a hard time expressing?

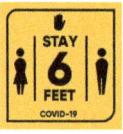
Who or what have you distanced yourself from that could help you overcome the above struggles/difficulties?

NEXT STEPS: Make a healthy plan of action that you will implement in order to help protect yourself from being overtaken by the daily stress of the pandemic. _____
_____
_____
_____
_____
_____
_____

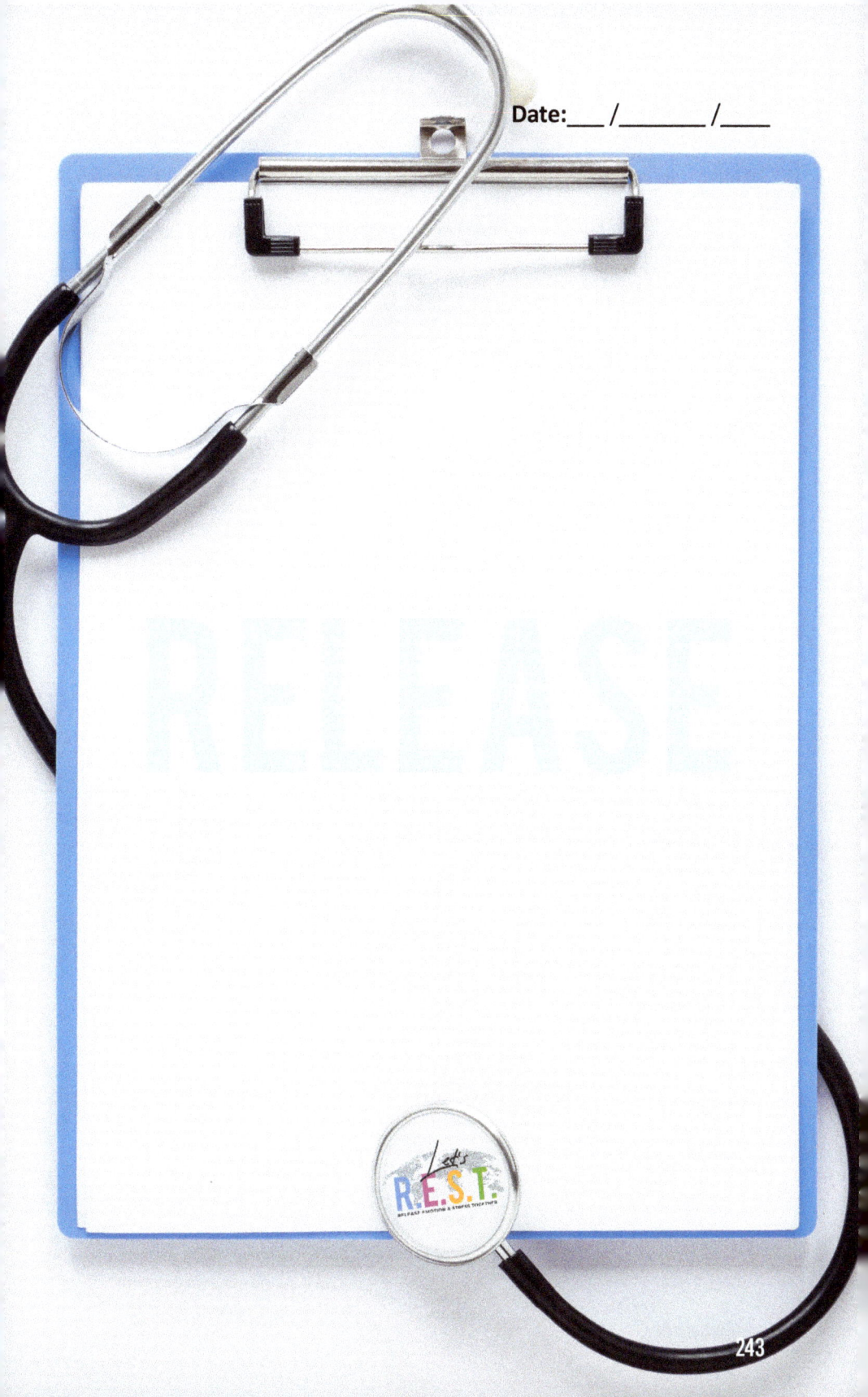

In order to seize our tomorrow, I believe that we must prepare today.
In preparation for tomorrow, I've discovered
that our todays give many lessons.
When we embrace the lessons of today, we are strengthened
emotionally and physically for our tomorrow.
Therefore, the victory for tomorrow is in the submitting to the
inner change and transformation from the lessons of our today.

— —Dr. Chevelta A. Smith

What did you learn **TODAY,** and *how* will you apply this knowledge to become a better/healthier you **TOMORROW?**

Let's R.E.S.T. **Bedtime Affirmation**
(Say it out loud!)

I am strong!
I am resilient!
I am able to overcome every disappointment and setback from today
I am more than a conqueror!
I will recharge myself with good sleep tonight
I will awake with a renewed sense of purpose
And I declare that my tomorrow will be great!

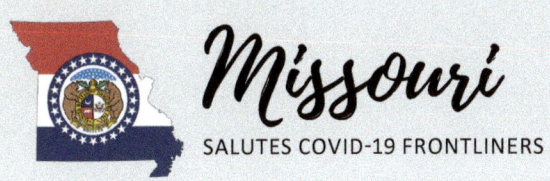

Missouri
SALUTES COVID-19 FRONTLINERS

The first responders have shown an extraordinary amount of courage during the COVID-19 pandemic. These brave individuals did not allow fear to grip their hearts, as the number of infected individuals exceeded 4M and the death toll beyond 600 K. The first responders should be rewarded for the long hours worked, pleasant demeanors, and exceptional skills to mitigate the destruction caused by the coronavirus.

—Rachel H.
St. Louis, Missouri

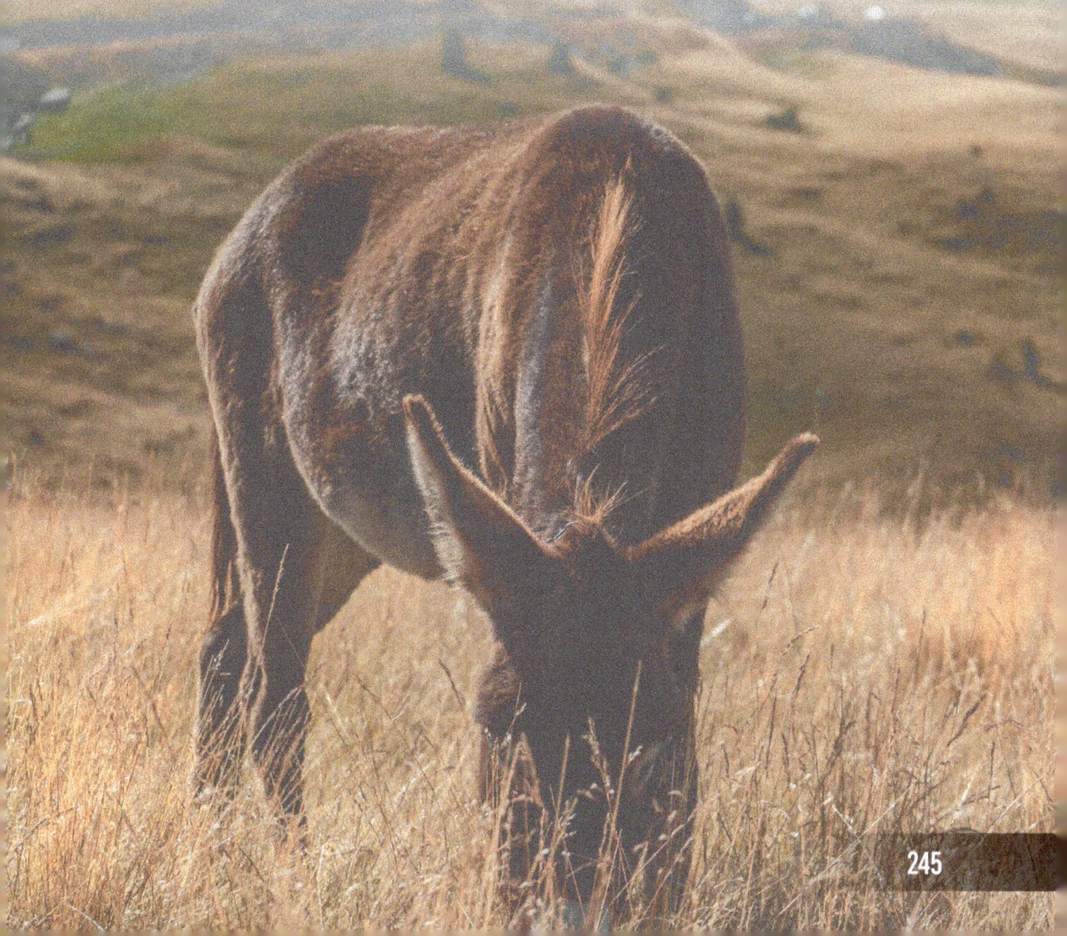

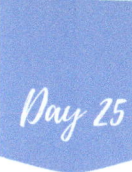

Day 25

MORNING HUDDLE

Not Only Are You Able to Complete Something, But You Can Complete It Well.

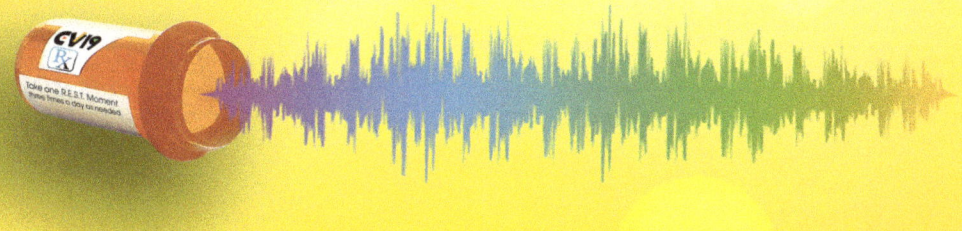

"You are able to deliver the greatness that is in you."
—Dr. Chevelta A. Smith

ABLE

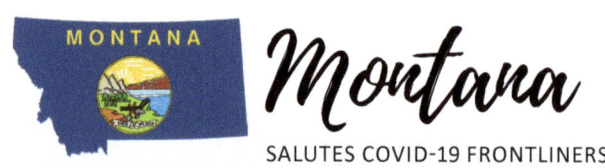

Montana

SALUTES COVID-19 FRONTLINERS

I see the frontline workers in the hospitals like I see soldiers -- there are things you will endure in the field that not many can say they've experienced, but they have the knowledge, ability, and know the job must be done. So they step up and are the heroes that say, "I'll go" without a hesitation. I can't imagine what they are going through, but I will forever thank them for passing as an essential frontline worker.
Thank you for everything you are doing!

—*Lawrence J. Atkins*
Lakeside, Montana

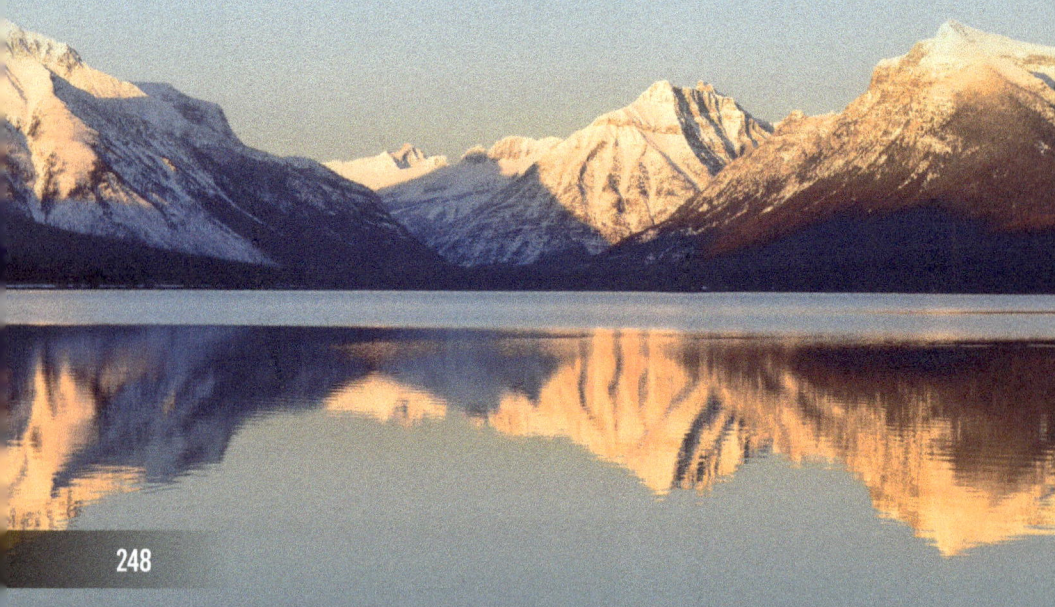

R

Today I RELEASED my... (check all that apply)

Mind By:
- ■ Communicating my thoughts, feelings, & needs to others
- ■ Speaking positive self-affirmations ■ Deep breathing ■ Other _____

Body By:
- ■ Muscle Relaxation Techniques ■ Exercise
- ■ Hydrotherapy: bath or shower ■ Other _____

Spirit By:
- ■ Meditation ■ Journaling ■ Praying
- ■ Going outside for 15-20 minutes ■ Self-Talk ■ Other _____

E

Today I FEEL... (circle one)

Happy / Anger / Love / Sad / Fear

Surprise / Disgust / Trust / Anticipation

Other _____

What is your dominant **EMOTION** in your life right now?

S

What were your main **STRESSORS** today?

What *Methods* are you using today **TO REDUCE** your current stress?

What *Value* have you noticed **IN USING** them?

T

Stick TOGETHER: How did you *Connect* today?

- ○ Reached out to a co-worker who appeared to be struggling
- ○ Expressed openly with trusted family or co-workers about how the pandemic is affecting me
- ○ Identified factors that are overwhelming/stressful and worked with others to find solutions
- ○ Initiated the "Buddy" System with other co-workers and monitored each other for signs of stress, burnout, and depression
- ○ Spoke to a mental health care provider

My ~~Let~~'s **R.E.S.T.** *Affirmation for Today:*
I will accomplish everything I need to do today. I am able to overcome every difficulty.

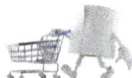

What do you need, but feel like it's unavailable?

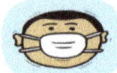

What are you having a hard time expressing?

Who or what have you distanced yourself from that could help you overcome the above struggles/difficulties?

NEXT STEPS: Make a healthy plan of action that you will implement in order to help protect yourself from being overtaken by the daily stress of the pandemic. _____
_____
_____
_____
_____
_____
_____

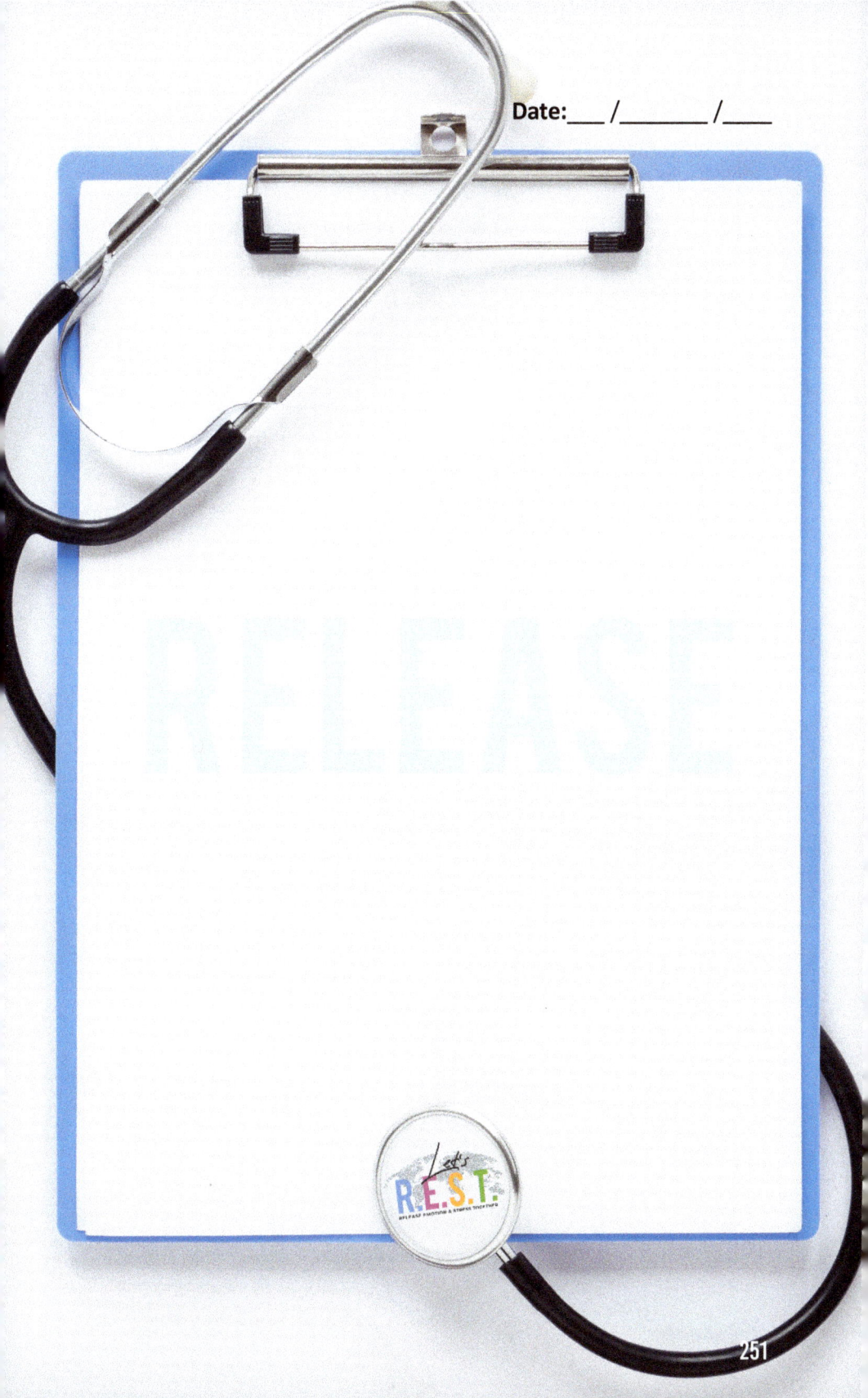

In order to seize our tomorrow, I believe that we must prepare today.
In preparation for tomorrow, I've discovered
that our todays give many lessons.
When we embrace the lessons of today, we are strengthened
emotionally and physically for our tomorrow.
Therefore, the victory for tomorrow is in the submitting to the
inner change and transformation from the lessons of our today.

--Dr. Chevelta A. Smith

What did you learn **TODAY**, and *how* will you apply this knowledge to become a better/healthier you **TOMORROW?**

Let's R.E.S.T. **Bedtime Affirmation**
(Say it out loud!)

I am strong!
I am resilient!
I am able to overcome every disappointment and setback from today
I am more than a conqueror!
I will recharge myself with good sleep tonight
I will awake with a renewed sense of purpose
And I declare that my tomorrow will be great!

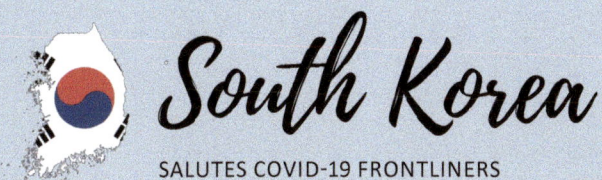
South Korea
SALUTES COVID-19 FRONTLINERS

우선, 코로나 19로 고생해주시는 의료진분들께 감사의 말씀을 드립니다.
그리고 제가 많은 도움을 드릴 수 없음에 죄송합니다.
간호사를 꿈꾸는 고등학생으로서, 의료진분들의 희생이 굉장히 대단하다고 생각했습니다.
감염의 위험이 있음에도 불구하고, 주저하지 않고 코로나 최전방에서 환자들을 돌
보는 여러분이 있었기에 전보다는 더 나아진 환경에서 살아갈 수 있는 것 같습니다.
그러면서 저 스스로 생각해보았습니다. '간호사가 되어 그러한 환경에 처하게 되면,
금의 의료진들처럼 용기있게 나서서 감염현장으로 나갈 수 있을까?'
그러나 선뜻 답변할 수 없었습니다. 모든이가 의료계의 외면은 그저 화려하고,
돈을 많이 버는 직업이라고 생각하겠지만 한편으론 매우 힘들고, 환자들
을 돌보느라 잠도 자지 못하는 환경에서 지내시는 것을 잘 알고있습니다
. 이런 생각을 하고나니, 수고해주시는 모든 의료진분들의 노고가 얼마나 용감하
고 대단한 것인지 깨달을 수 있었습니다. 모든 의료진분들은 우리의 영웅입니다.
하루빨리 코로나19 사태가 끝나 모든 사람들이 마스크 없이 행복했으면 좋겠습니다.
그 누가 여러분의 노고를 알지 못하더라도, 너무 힘들어서 포기해버리고 싶을지라도,
가 마지막 단 한 사람이 되어 여러분의 그 힘듦을 알아드리겠습니다.
제가 있는 이 자리에서 최선을 다하겠습니다. 항상 감사하고, 존경합니다!

윤수진
(인천, 한국)

(English Translation):
First of all, I would like to thank the medical workers who are suffering from COVID-19. And I feel sorry that I can't help you more. As a high school student who dreams of being a nurse in the future, I thought that the sacrifices of all you guys were great.
We can live in safer circumstances thanks to your hard work, which is sent to the frontline of the virus and takes care of the patients without any hesitation despite the high risk of infection. So, I just thought to myself, seeing your hard work, 'what if I am in this situation when I become a nurse? Can I go to the frontline of the virus bravely like they did?' But I couldn't answer readily. Also, even though people think that the medical industries would earn much money and look so fancy, I do know that working in the medical industry is not easy. And you can't even get much sleep when you're so busy taking care of the patients. With all these thoughts, I realized how you are brave and amazing. What can I possibly say more about your sacrifice? You are our hero.
I want COVID-19 to end as soon as possible and people from the entire world would be happy without a mask. Even if everyone isn't aware of your hard work or it's too hard so that you want to give up, I will be the person who knows and supports your hard work for this situation. I will do my best here. I appreciate you all the time and respect you!

—Yoon Su Jin
(Incheon, Korea)

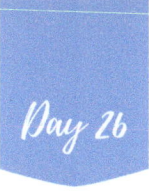

Day 26

MORNING HUDDLE

You Are Encouraged to Pray for Your Day, Before You Even Begin It.

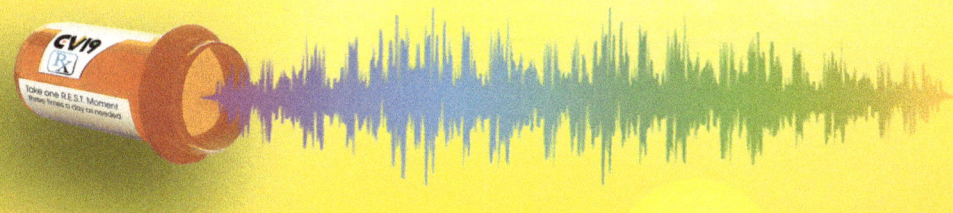

"Pray for your day."
—Dr. Chevelta A. Smith

PRAY

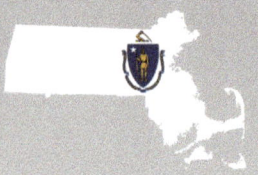

Massachusetts
SALUTES COVID-19 FRONTLINERS

God, who calls all humanity to serve -- You've called healthcare workers to their profession to heal and to save. You've gifted them so that they might bring their best training and experience to bear. Receive the pain they feel despite their best efforts, and when they watch countless people die. You are the God who heals the broken-hearted (Psalm 147:3). So, shield their hearts from undue pain so that they, in turn, may console each other). Amen!

Thank you will never be enough for what you do. Stay strong and know that there are people all over our great nation praying for you.

*—Christina Anop,
Cape Cod, Massachusetts*

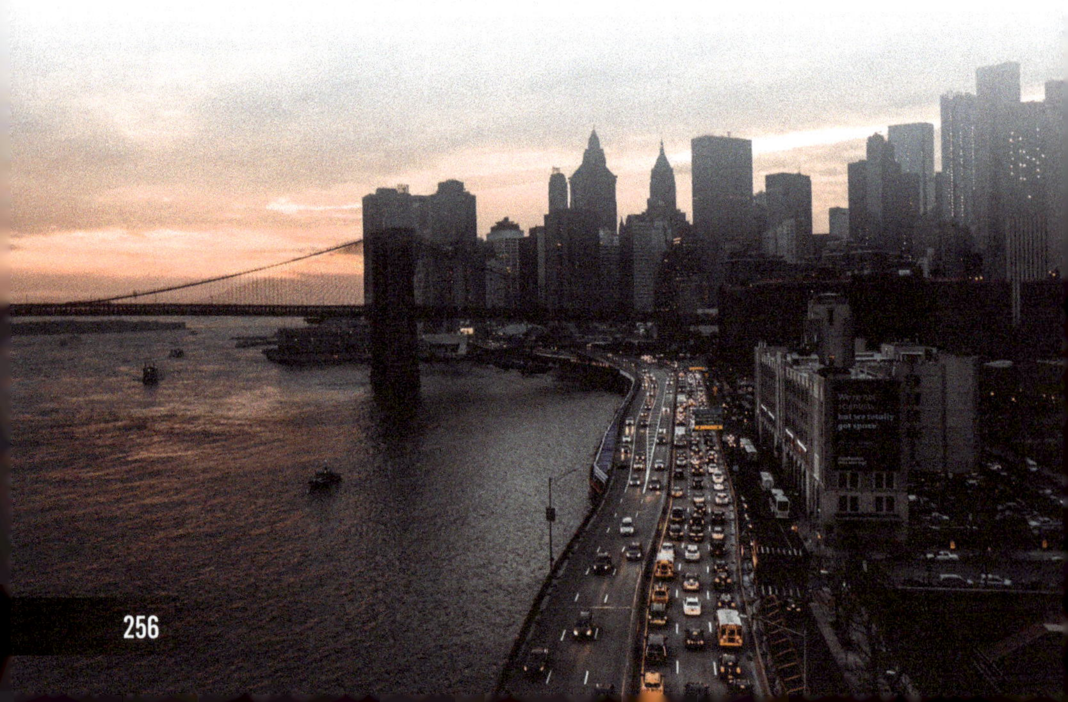

R

Today I RELEASED my... *(check all that apply)*

Mind By:
- Communicating my thoughts, feelings, & needs to others
- Speaking positive self-affirmations
- Deep breathing
- Other _____

Body By:
- Muscle Relaxation Techniques
- Exercise
- Hydrotherapy: bath or shower
- Other _____

Spirit By:
- Meditation
- Journaling
- Praying
- Going outside for 15-20 minutes
- Self-Talk
- Other _____

E

Today I FEEL... *(circle one)*

Happy / Anger / Love / Sad / Fear

Surprise / Disgust / Trust / Anticipation

Other _____

What is your dominant EMOTION in your life right now?

S

What were your main STRESSORS today?

What Methods are you using today TO REDUCE your current stress?

What Value have you noticed IN USING them?

T

Stick TOGETHER: How did you Connect today?

- Reached out to a co-worker who appeared to be struggling
- Expressed openly with trusted family or co-workers about how the pandemic is affecting me
- Identified factors that are overwhelming/stressful and worked with others to find solutions
- Initiated the "Buddy" System with other co-workers and monitored each other for signs of stress, burnout, and depression
- Spoke to a mental health care provider

My Led's R.E.S.T. Affirmation for Today:

Today I pray that I am blessed and my day is blessed! I will have the ability to manage every task set before me. Today will be a great day!

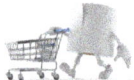 What do you need, but feel like it's unavailable?

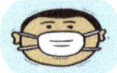 What are you having a hard time expressing?

 Who or what have you distanced yourself from that could help you overcome the above struggles/difficulties?

 NEXT STEPS: Make a healthy plan of action that you will implement in order to help protect yourself from being overtaken by the daily stress of the pandemic. _____
_____
_____
_____
_____
_____
_____

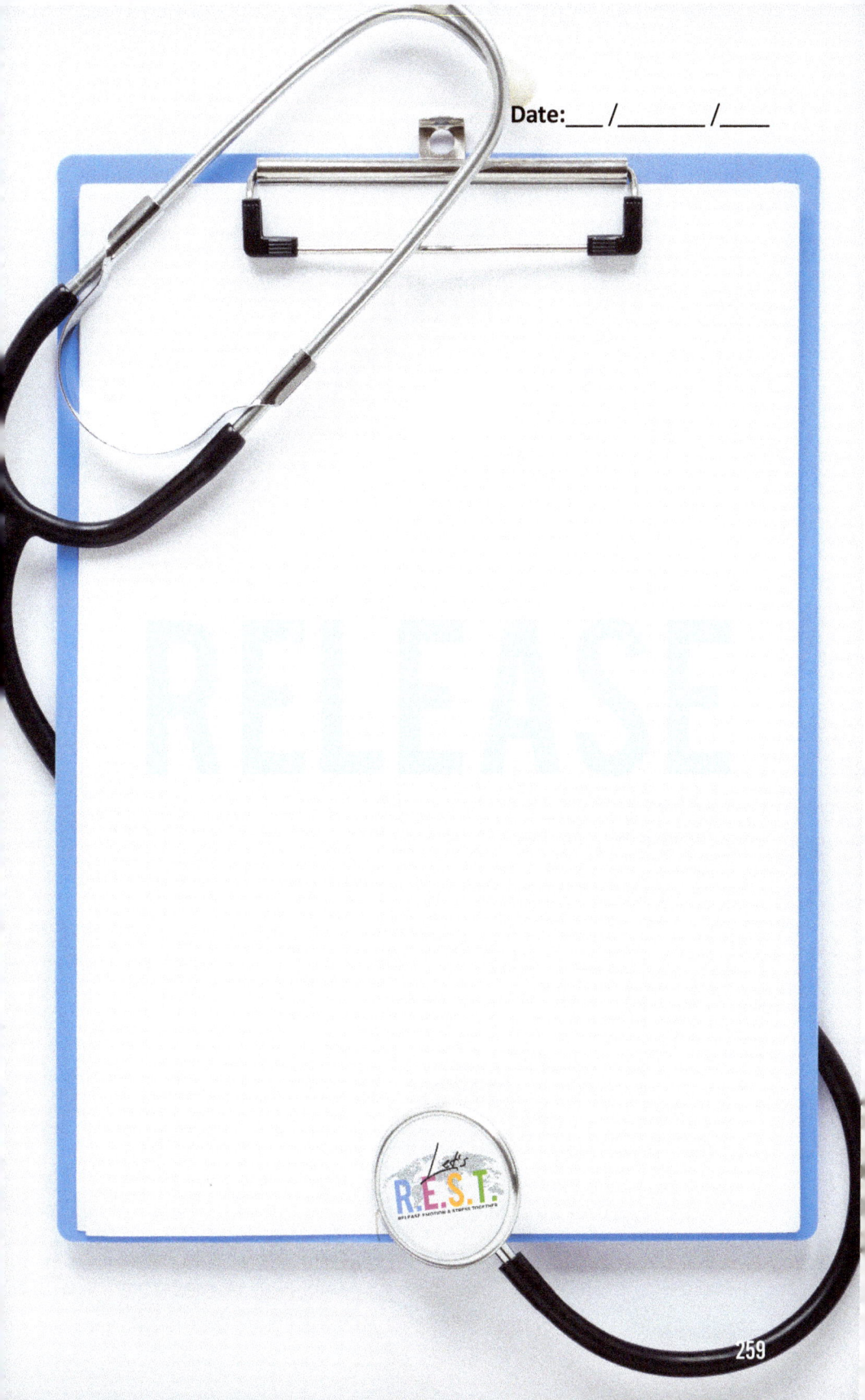

In order to seize our tomorrow, I believe that we must prepare today.
In preparation for tomorrow, I've discovered
that our todays give many lessons.
When we embrace the lessons of today, we are strengthened
emotionally and physically for our tomorrow.
Therefore, the victory for tomorrow is in the submitting to the
inner change and transformation from the lessons of our today.

—–Dr. Chevelta A. Smith

> *What* did you learn **TODAY**, and *how* will you apply this knowledge to become a better/healthier you **TOMORROW?**

Let's R.E.S.T. **Bedtime Affirmation**
(Say it out loud!)

I am strong!
I am resilient!
I am able to overcome every disappointment and setback from today
I am more than a conqueror!
I will recharge myself with good sleep tonight
I will awake with a renewed sense of purpose
And I declare that my tomorrow will be great!

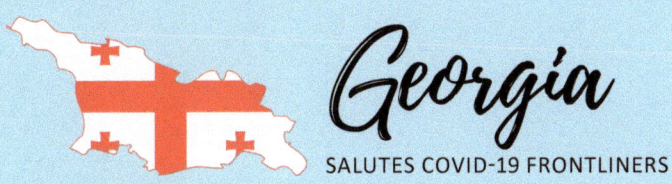
Georgia
SALUTES COVID-19 FRONTLINERS

Thank you ALL for the selflessness given each day.
Every day, alone or with others, read and believe the 91st Psalms.
God will protect you.

—Lorene Smalls Brewer
Sylvania, Georgia

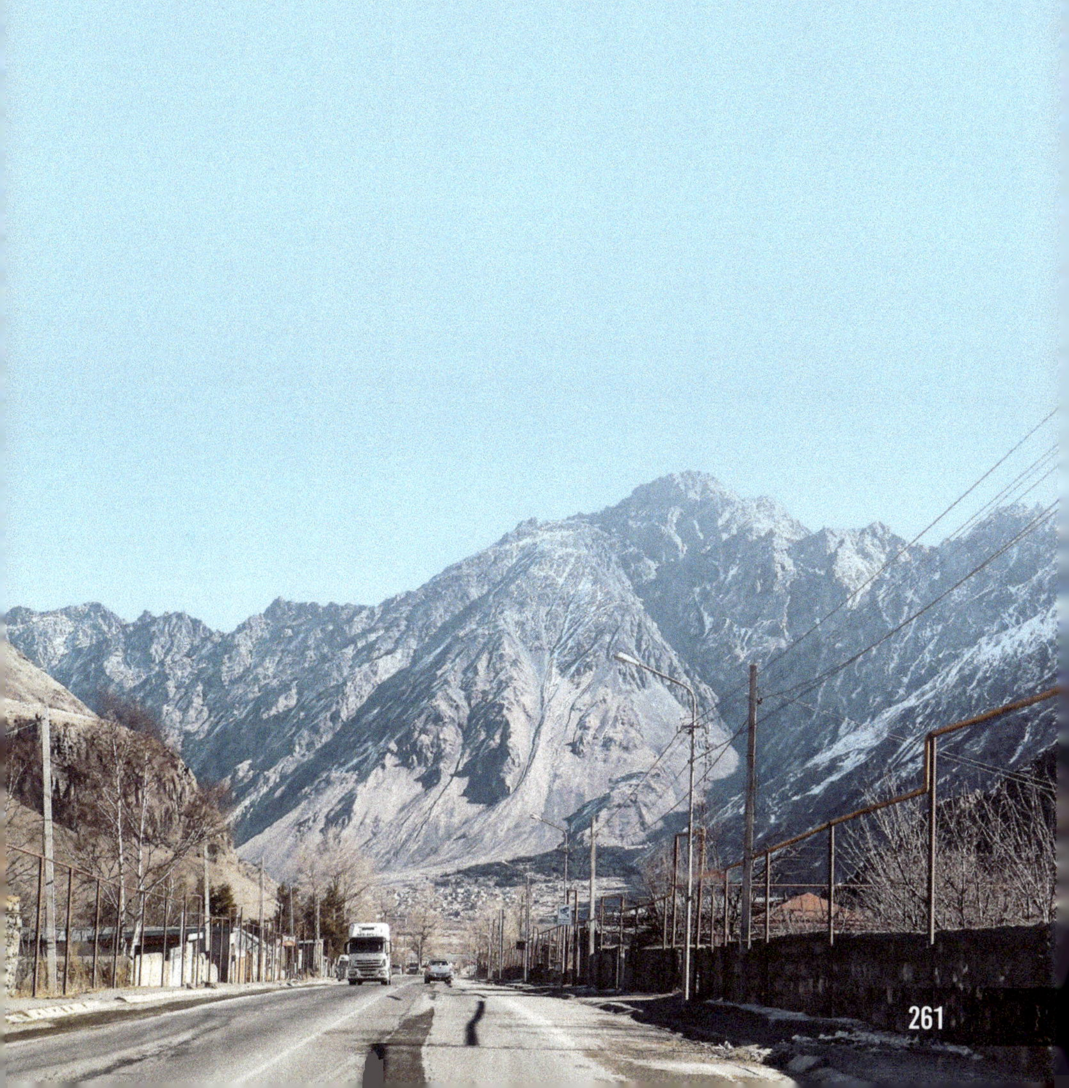

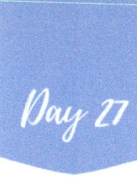

Day 27

MORNING HUDDLE

Have Faith In Yourself That You Can Do Whatever You Desire to Do.

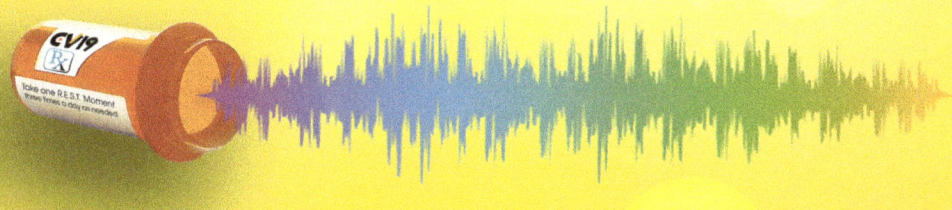

Fear always seeks to demolish faith. So, you have to learn to tell fear to —Shut Up!"

—Dr. Chevelta A. Smith

FAITH

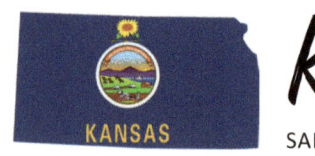 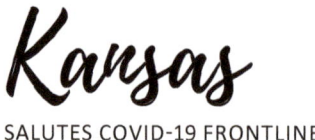

Kansas
SALUTES COVID-19 FRONTLINERS

As we continue to move forward during this time of COVID-19, we encourage everyone to stay home whenever possible. However, there are unsung heroes who must every day face the realities of contracting this virus that they may never recover from.

Every day you wrap yourselves in faith and go to serve others. Thank you seems so small, and yet is the most powerful expression I have. I salute all the frontline workers and lend my continued prayers and support.

—Pastor Aaron H. Henson
Kansas City, Kansas

R

Today I RELEASED my... (check all that apply)

Mind By:
- ■ Communicating my thoughts, feelings, & needs to others
- ■ Speaking positive self-affirmations ■ Deep breathing ■ Other _____

Body By:
- ■ Muscle Relaxation Techniques   ■ Exercise
- ■ Hydrotherapy: bath or shower   ■ Other _____

Spirit By:
- ■ Meditation   ■ Journaling   ■ Praying
- ■ Going outside for 15-20 minutes   ■ Self-Talk   ■ Other _____

E

Today I FEEL... (circle one)

Happy / Anger / Love / Sad / Fear

Surprise / Disgust / Trust / Anticipation

Other_____

What is your dominant **EMOTION** in your life right now?

S

What were your main **STRESSORS** today?

What *Methods* are you using today **TO REDUCE** your current stress?

What *Value* have you noticed **IN USING** them?

T

Stick TOGETHER: How did you *Connect* today?

- ○ Reached out to a co-worker who appeared to be struggling
- ○ Expressed openly with trusted family or co-workers about how the pandemic is affecting me
- ○ Identified factors that are overwhelming/stressful and worked with others to find solutions
- ○ Initiated the "Buddy" System with other co-workers and monitored each other for signs of stress, burnout, and depression
- ○ Spoke to a mental health care provider

My *Let's* R.E.S.T. *Affirmation for Today:*
I believe in myself! I have faith in my ability to achieve my dreams and goals.

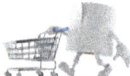 What do you need, but feel like it's unavailable?

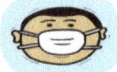 What are you having a hard time expressing?

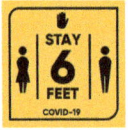 Who or what have you distanced yourself from that could help you overcome the above struggles/difficulties?

 NEXT STEPS: Make a healthy plan of action that you will implement in order to help protect yourself from being overtaken by the daily stress of the pandemic. _____
_____
_____
_____
_____
_____

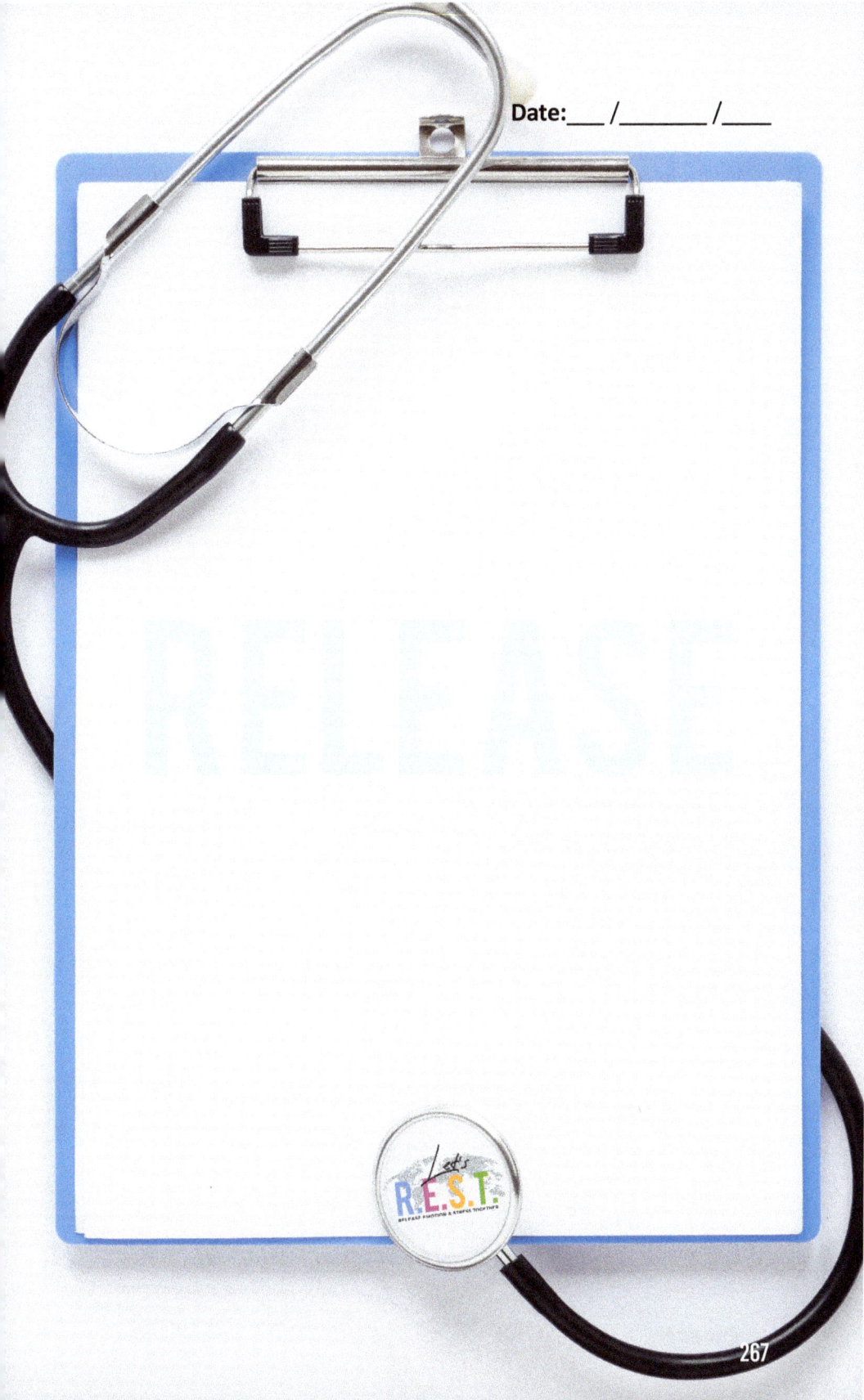

Date:___ / _____ / ___

In order to seize our tomorrow, I believe that we must prepare today.
In preparation for tomorrow, I've discovered
that our todays give many lessons.
When we embrace the lessons of today, we are strengthened
emotionally and physically for our tomorrow.
Therefore, the victory for tomorrow is in the submitting to the
inner change and transformation from the lessons of our today.

--Dr. Chevelta A. Smith

What did you learn **TODAY**, and *how* will you apply this knowledge to become a better/healthier you **TOMORROW?**

Let's R.E.S.T. Bedtime Affirmation
(Say it out loud!)

I am strong!
I am resilient!
I am able to overcome every disappointment and setback from today
I am more than a conqueror!
I will recharge myself with good sleep tonight
I will awake with a renewed sense of purpose
And I declare that my tomorrow will be great!

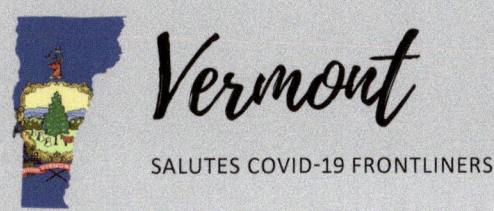

Vermont

SALUTES COVID-19 FRONTLINERS

Thank you for your unwavering fight against this demon that is COVID-19. Your selflessness is humbling.

—Heather B.
Weston, Vermont

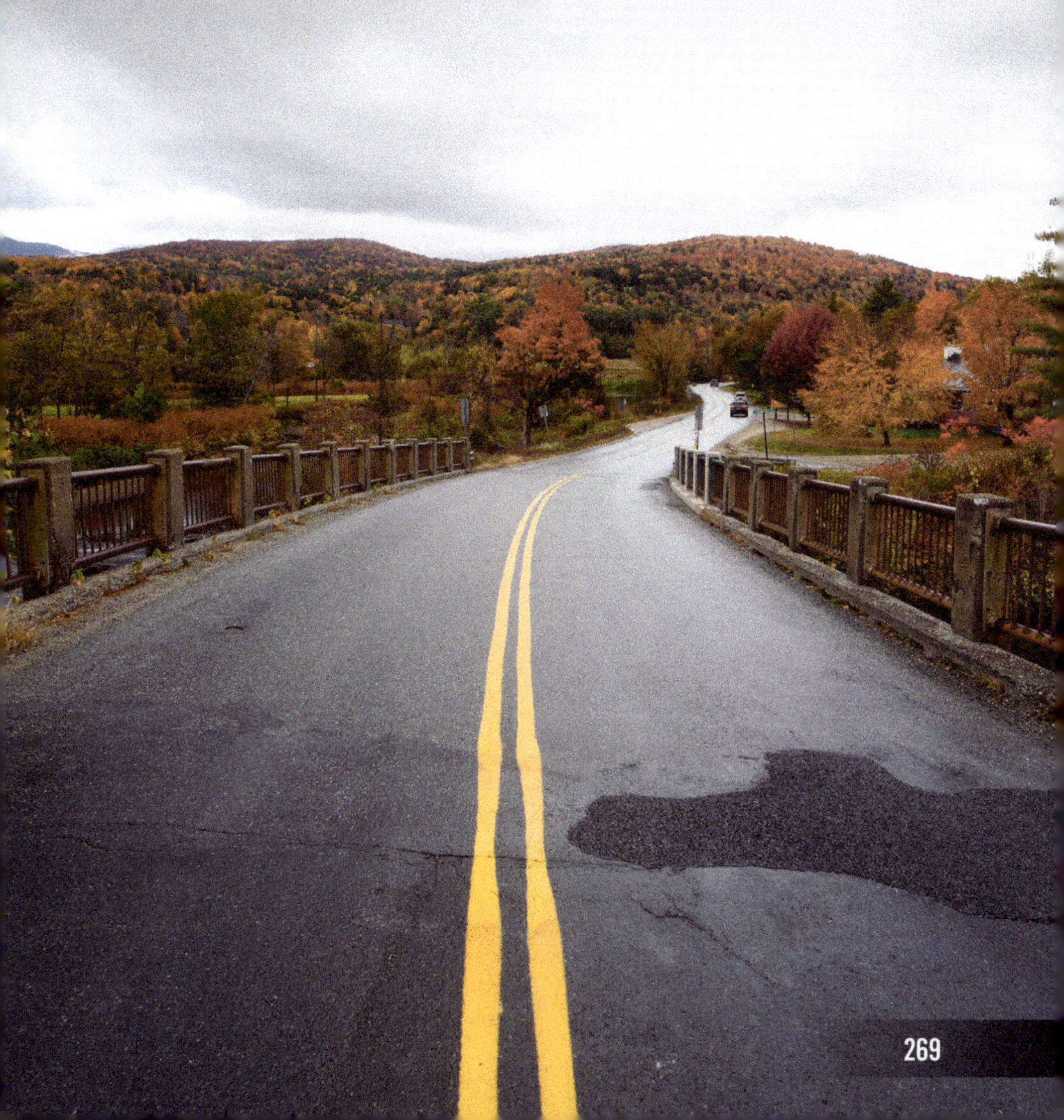

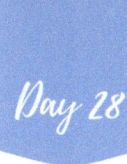

Day 28

MORNING HUDDLE

You're Worthy of Success! You're Worthy of Joy! You're Worthy to Be Financially Blessed! You're Worthy to Be Healed and Whole in Your Life.

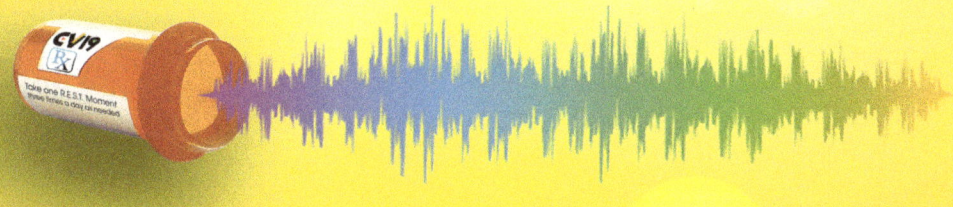

"Don't doubt you're worthy—cash in on yourself!"
—Dr. Chevelta A. Smith

AFFIRMATION WORTHY 2

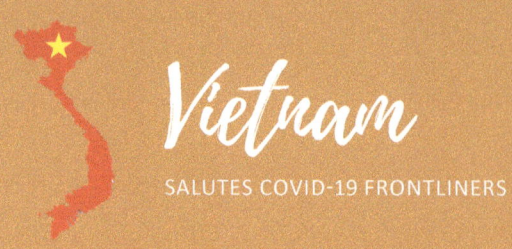

Vietnam
SALUTES COVID-19 FRONTLINERS

Cảmơnnhữngngườigiúpđỡnhữngngườibệnhtronglúcnguyhiểm. Khôngcónhữngngườinhưvậythìcảthếgiớicùngnhauđauđớn!

English translation:
Thank you to all the people who are helping patients in these dangerous times. Without you, the whole world would be suffering much more collectively.

—Anonymous from Vietnam

R

Today **I RELEASED** *my*... *(check all that apply)*

Mind By:
- Communicating my thoughts, feelings, & needs to others
- Speaking positive self-affirmations
- Deep breathing
- Other _____

Body By:
- Muscle Relaxation Techniques
- Exercise
- Hydrotherapy: bath or shower
- Other _____

Spirit By:
- Meditation
- Journaling
- Praying
- Going outside for 15-20 minutes
- Self-Talk
- Other _____

E

Today **I FEEL**... *(circle one)*

Happy / Anger / Love / Sad / Fear

Surprise / Disgust / Trust / Anticipation

Other _____

What is your dominant **EMOTION** in your life right now?

S

What were your main **STRESSORS** today?

What *Methods* are you using today **TO REDUCE** your current stress?

What *Value* have you noticed **IN USING** them?

T

Stick **TOGETHER**: How did you *Connect* today?

- Reached out to a co-worker who appeared to be struggling
- Expressed openly with trusted family or co-workers about how the pandemic is affecting me
- Identified factors that are overwhelming/stressful and worked with others to find solutions
- Initiated the "Buddy" System with other co-workers and monitored each other for signs of stress, burnout, and depression
- Spoke to a mental health care provider

My *Let's* R.E.S.T. *Affirmation for Today:*
I am worthy of good things coming in my life. I have value.

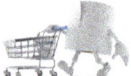 What do you need, but feel like it's unavailable?

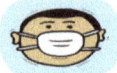 What are you having a hard time expressing?

 Who or what have you distanced yourself from that could help you overcome the above struggles/difficulties?

 **NEXT STEPS: Make a healthy plan of action that you will implement in order to help protect yourself from being overtaken by the daily stress of the pandemic.** _____

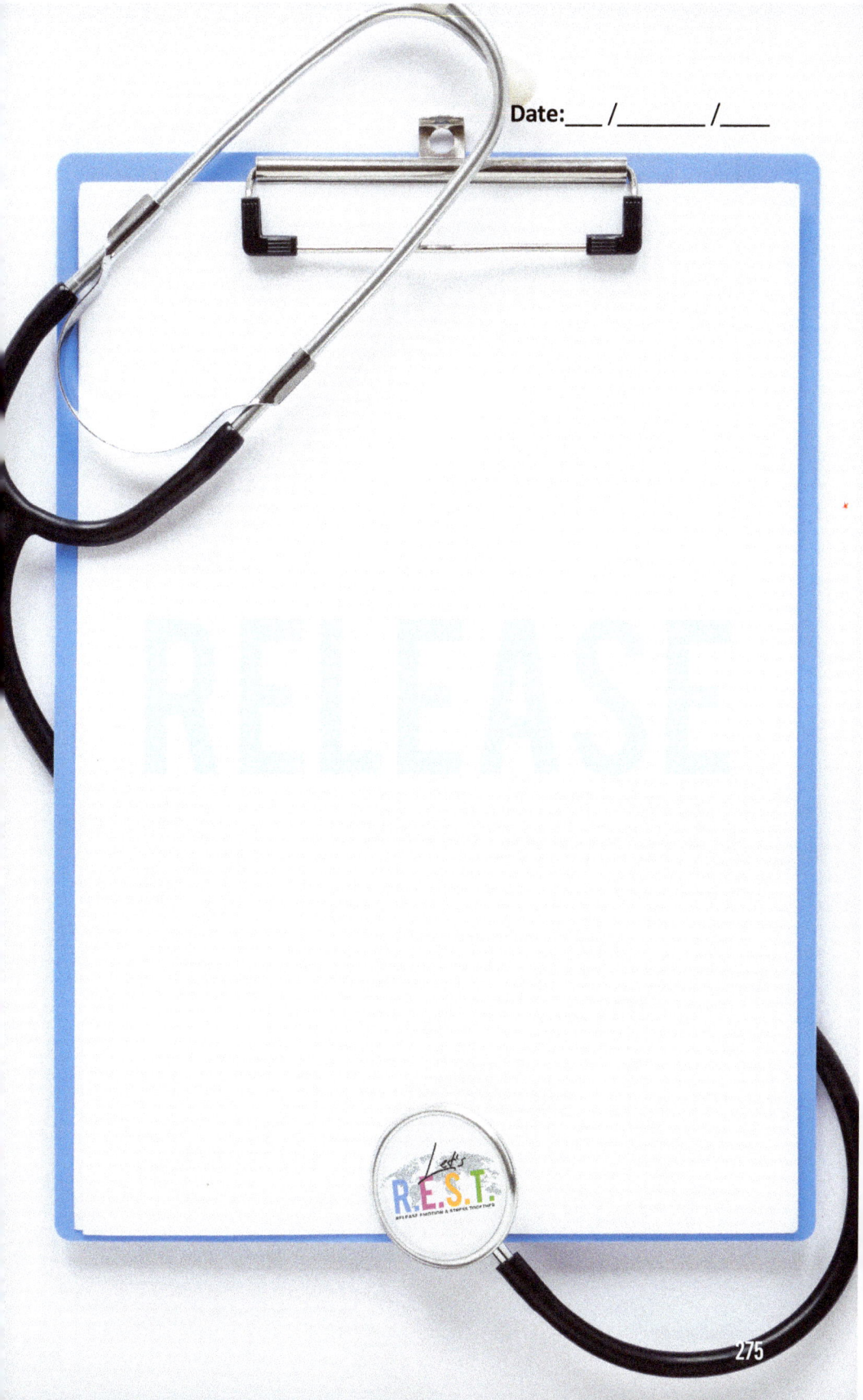

In order to seize our tomorrow, I believe that we must prepare today.
In preparation for tomorrow, I've discovered
that our todays give many lessons.
When we embrace the lessons of today, we are strengthened
emotionally and physically for our tomorrow.
Therefore, the victory for tomorrow is in the submitting to the
inner change and transformation from the lessons of our today.

--Dr. Chevelta A. Smith

What did you learn **TODAY**, and *how* will you apply this knowledge to become a better/healthier you **TOMORROW?**

Let's R.E.S.T. **Bedtime Affirmation**
(Say it out loud!)

I am strong!
I am resilient!
I am able to overcome every disappointment and setback from today
I am more than a conqueror!
I will recharge myself with good sleep tonight
I will awake with a renewed sense of purpose
And I declare that my tomorrow will be great!

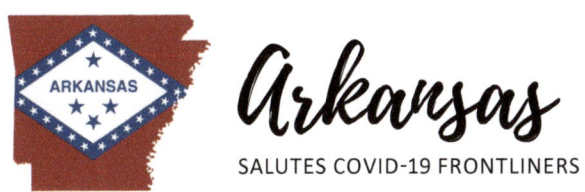

Arkansas
SALUTES COVID-19 FRONTLINERS

I wish I could send you the strength to get through this. Many of us are doing all we can not to put your life at risk. Keep up the good fight! We are so blessed to have people like you who put your fellow citizens first. You are the true heroes.

—DM Bridgette D. Thomas.
Osceola, Arkansas

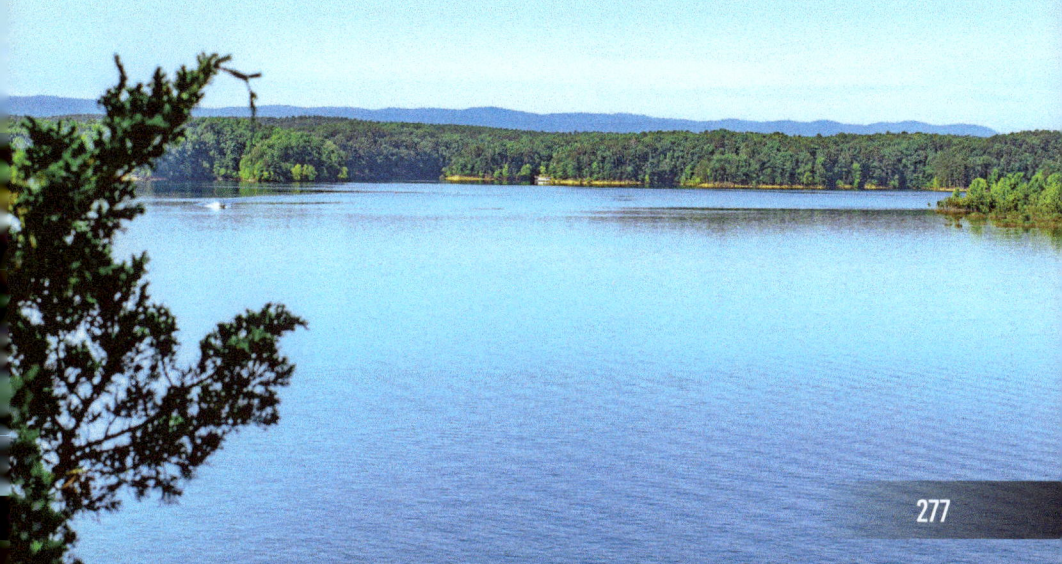

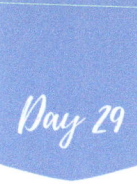

MORNING HUDDLE

There Is Often a Process That Has to Take Place to Lead Us to the Progress That We are Anticipating to Receive. Be Patient, You Will Complete the Process.

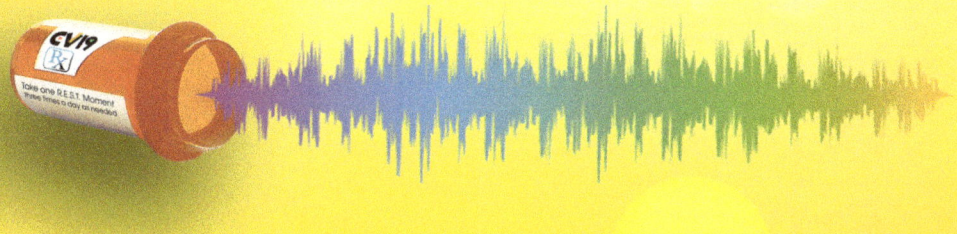

"Faith is knowing that you are going to be okay."
—Dr. Chevelta A. Smith

FAITH TO KNOW

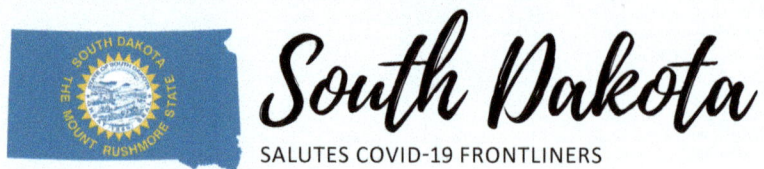

South Dakota

SALUTES COVID-19 FRONTLINERS

To our frontline workers during this COVID-19 pandemic: Know that this immeasurable feat you've undertaken and the selflessness with which you've faced it reflect the true nature of God. A God who understands that anxiety and fear will surface but you can trust that "When you pass through the waters, He will be with you; and through the rivers, they shall not overwhelm you; when you walk through fire you shall not be burned, and the flame shall not consume you"- Isaiah 43:2. Even in the midst of death and sickness, be assured that He is God from beginning to the end and His love for you will never fail. Know that He sees you, He sees your sacrifice, and He knows your name.

So, to our unsung heroes--the healthcare workers, pharmacists, mail carriers, food delivery drivers, grocery store employees, and others who are keeping us safe and fed and cared for, please remember after the battle; the reward: the reward of knowing your sacrifice will never be in vain,"Therefore, my beloved brothers, be steadfast, immovable, always abounding in the work of the Lord, knowing that in the Lord your labor is not in vain."-1 Corinthians 15:58

*—Anthonette M.
South Dakota*

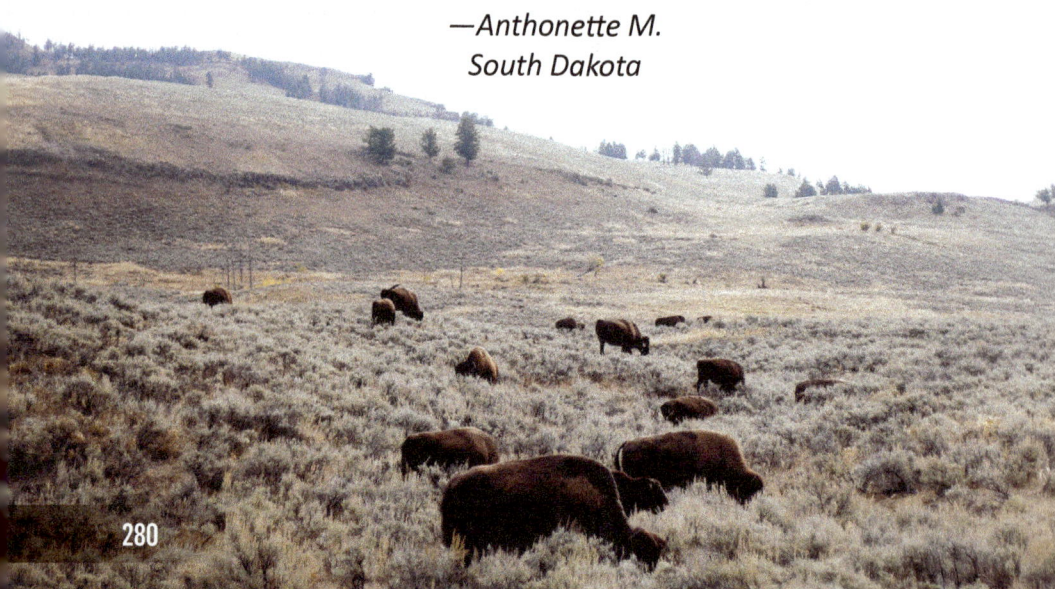

R

Today I RELEASED my... (check all that apply)

Mind By:
- ■ Communicating my thoughts, feelings, & needs to others
- ■ Speaking positive self-affirmations   ■ Deep breathing   ■ Other _____

Body By:
- ■ Muscle Relaxation Techniques   ■ Exercise
- ■ Hydrotherapy: bath or shower   ■ Other _____

Spirit By:
- ■ Meditation   ■ Journaling   ■ Praying
- ■ Going outside for 15-20 minutes   ■ Self-Talk   ■ Other _____

E

Today I FEEL... (circle one)

Happy / Anger / Love / Sad / Fear

Surprise / Disgust / Trust / Anticipation

Other _____

What is your dominant **EMOTION** in your life right now?

S

What were your main **STRESSORS** today?

What *Methods* are you using today **TO REDUCE** your current stress?

What *Value* have you noticed **IN USING** them?

T

Stick TOGETHER: How did you *Connect* today?

- Reached out to a co-worker who appeared to be struggling
- Expressed openly with trusted family or co-workers about how the pandemic is affecting me
- Identified factors that are overwhelming/stressful and worked with others to find solutions
- Initiated the "Buddy" System with other co-workers and monitored each other for signs of stress, burnout, and depression
- Spoke to a mental health care provider

My *Let's* **R.E.S.T.** *Affirmation for Today:*

I will have the faith to know that everything is going to be okay today, tomorrow, and in the many days ahead.

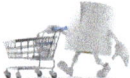 What do you need, but feel like it's unavailable?

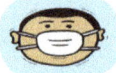 What are you having a hard time expressing?

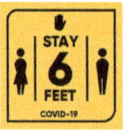 Who or what have you distanced yourself from that could help you overcome the above struggles/difficulties?

 **NEXT STEPS:** Make a healthy plan of action that you will implement in order to help protect yourself from being overtaken by the daily stress of the pandemic. _____
_____
_____
_____
_____
_____
_____

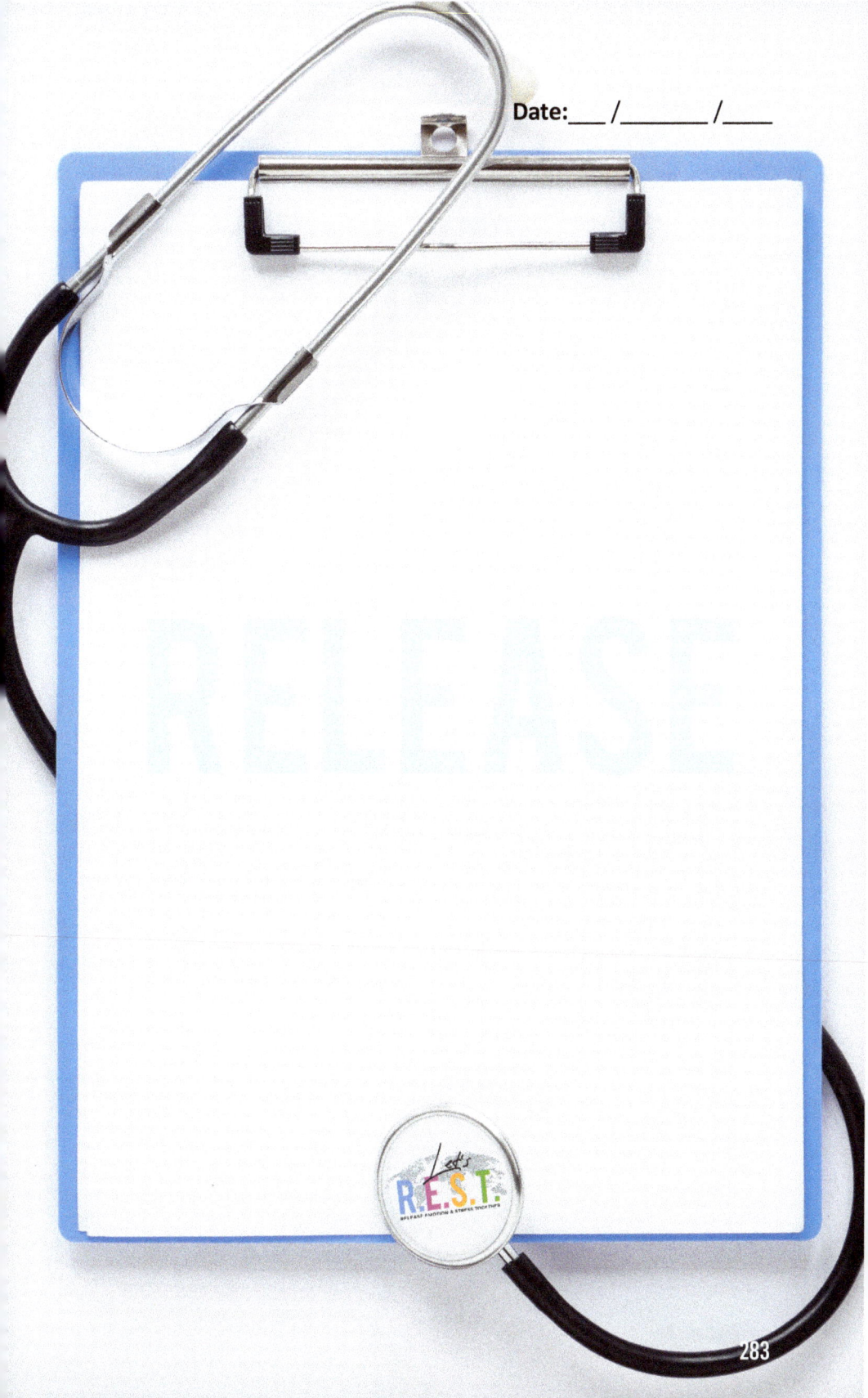

Date:___ /_____ /___

RELEASE

In order to seize our tomorrow, I believe that we must prepare today.
In preparation for tomorrow, I've discovered
that our todays give many lessons.
When we embrace the lessons of today, we are strengthened
emotionally and physically for our tomorrow.
Therefore, the victory for tomorrow is in the submitting to the
inner change and transformation from the lessons of our today.

--Dr. Chevelta A. Smith

What did you learn **TODAY**, and *how* will you apply this knowledge to become a better/healthier you **TOMORROW?**

Let's R.E.S.T. **Bedtime Affirmation**
(Say it out loud!)

I am strong!
I am resilient!
I am able to overcome every disappointment and setback from today
I am more than a conqueror!
I will recharge myself with good sleep tonight
I will awake with a renewed sense of purpose
And I declare that my tomorrow will be great!

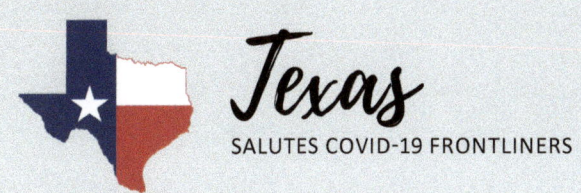

Texas
SALUTES COVID-19 FRONTLINERS

I have come to view [you] our medical workers on the frontlines the same way soldiers are viewed. While you all did not sign up for war, you are the ones fighting the battle to keep this nation safe. I hate the fact that in some ways, you are protecting us from ourselves. The fact that the most intelligent of us are battling ignorance, as well as an unseen enemy, seems fitting, but the cost often too high. I pray that those who read this know that your sacrifices are appreciated. Your stories need to be told. You are loved by this nation and are inspiring others.

*—William R.
Abilene, Texas*

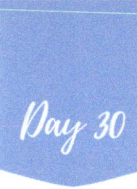

Day 30

MORNING HUDDLE

Being Great Does Not Mean That You Haven't Made Mistakes in Your Life. Being Great Does Not Mean That You Haven't Had Some Failures in Life. You're Great Because You Are Making a Difference in the Lives of Others.

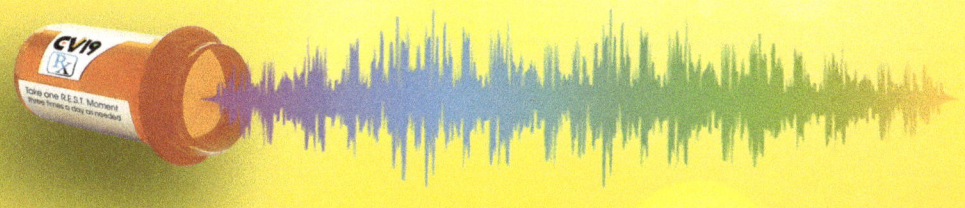

"It's our setbacks and upsets in life that are simply our setups for victory and greatness!"
—Dr. Chevelta A. Smith

GREAT

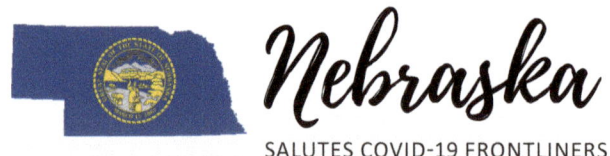

Nebraska
SALUTES COVID-19 FRONTLINERS

To every first responder, to every woman and man on the frontline, you are the heartbeat and rhythm of excellence. Your skilled hands, expedient feet, learned minds, and open hearts are the very source of what makes this world great. The cure and the solution to this time and season we are in shall be infinitely shortened and pronounced because you made your divine purpose for existence loud and clear. No words can adequately articulate your greatness but THANK YOU.

—Daemon S.
Nebraska

R

Today I RELEASED my... *(check all that apply)*

Mind By:
- Communicating my thoughts, feelings, & needs to others
- Speaking positive self-affirmations
- Deep breathing
- Other _____

Body By:
- Muscle Relaxation Techniques
- Exercise
- Hydrotherapy: bath or shower
- Other _____

Spirit By:
- Meditation
- Journaling
- Praying
- Going outside for 15-20 minutes
- Self-Talk
- Other _____

E

Today I FEEL... *(circle one)*

Happy / Anger / Love / Sad / Fear

Surprise / Disgust / Trust / Anticipation

Other_____

What is your dominant **EMOTION** in your life right now?

S

What were your main **STRESSORS** today?

What *Methods* are you using today **TO REDUCE** your current stress?

What *Value* have you noticed **IN USING** them?

T

Stick TOGETHER: How did you *Connect* today?

- Reached out to a co-worker who appeared to be struggling
- Expressed openly with trusted family or co-workers about how the pandemic is affecting me
- Identified factors that are overwhelming/stressful and worked with others to find solutions
- Initiated the "Buddy" System with other co-workers and monitored each other for signs of stress, burnout, and depression
- Spoke to a mental health care provider

My *Let's* R.E.S.T. *Affirmation for Today:*
I am great. I was born to be great!

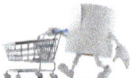
What do you need, but feel like it's unavailable?

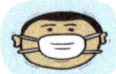
What are you having a hard time expressing?

Who or what have you distanced yourself from that could help you overcome the above struggles/difficulties?

NEXT STEPS: Make a healthy plan of action that you will implement in order to help protect yourself from being overtaken by the daily stress of the pandemic. _____
_____
_____
_____
_____
_____
_____

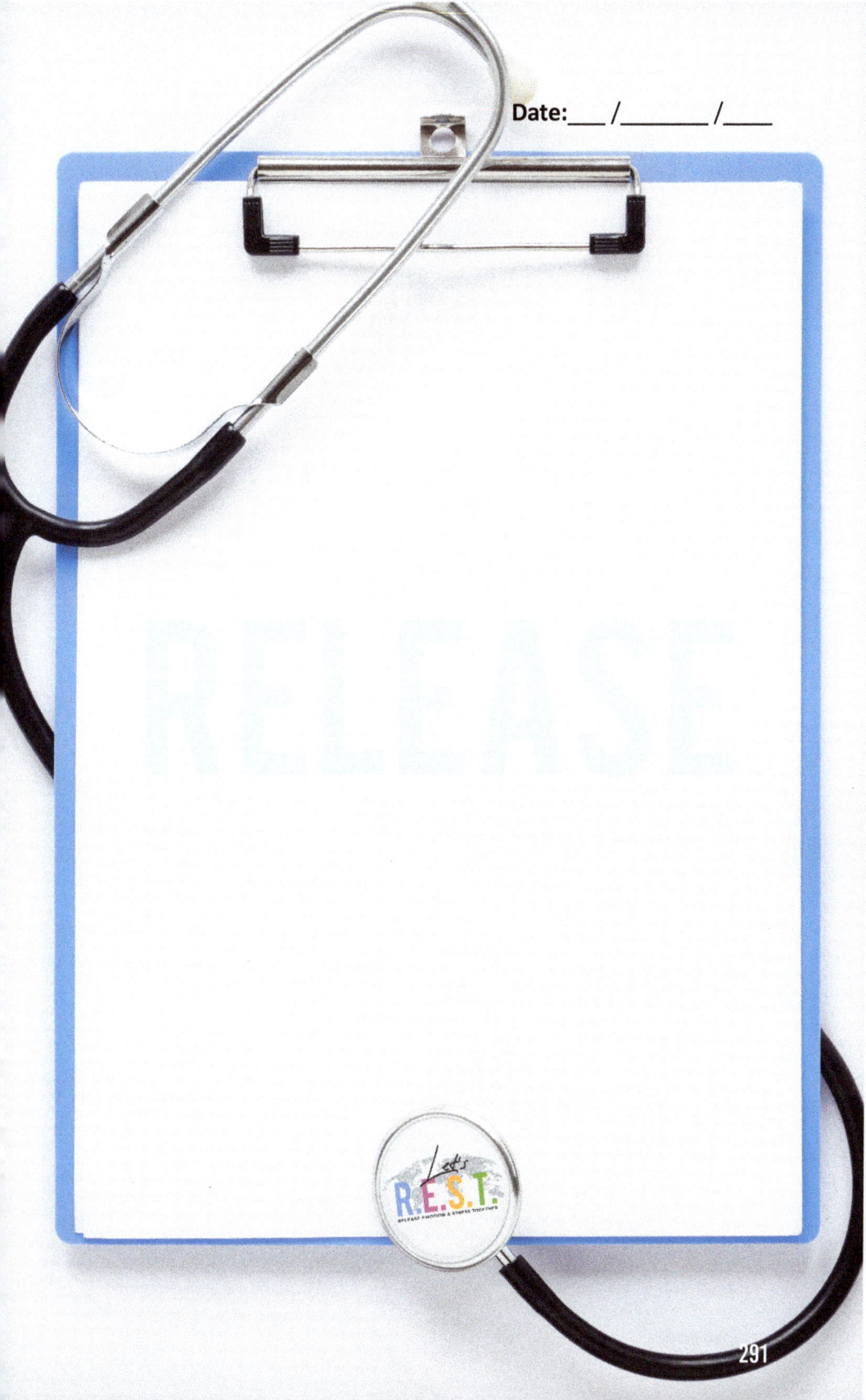

In order to seize our tomorrow, I believe that we must prepare today.
In preparation for tomorrow, I've discovered
that our todays give many lessons.
When we embrace the lessons of today, we are strengthened
emotionally and physically for our tomorrow.
Therefore, the victory for tomorrow is in the submitting to the
inner change and transformation from the lessons of our today.

--Dr. Chevelta A. Smith

What did you learn **TODAY**, and *how* will you apply this knowledge to become a better/healthier you **TOMORROW?**

Let's R.E.S.T. **Bedtime Affirmation**
(Say it out loud!)

I am strong!
I am resilient!
I am able to overcome every disappointment and setback from today
I am more than a conqueror!
I will recharge myself with good sleep tonight
I will awake with a renewed sense of purpose
And I declare that my tomorrow will be great!

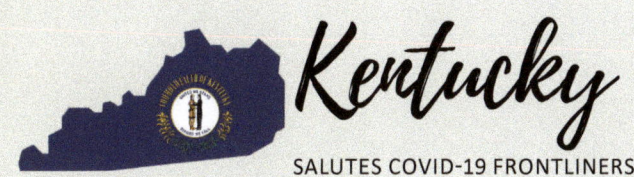

Kentucky

SALUTES COVID-19 FRONTLINERS

As a resident of Kentucky, I would like to extend thanks to all medical frontliner teams in all departments throughout the system for working tirelessly to take care of our community and us. Words cannot express how grateful we are to you for all that you have done for us. You have gone "Beyond the call of Duty;" you have put your life on the line to help us; and we just want to say, Thank You.

We thank you and stand with all of the doctors, nurses, technicians, support staff, frontliners, and all of you. Thank you for rising to the challenge and staying the course to get us well and keeping us well. Thank you for speaking up and speaking out about what we should and should not do. You have become family and, are in our prayers. Please stay safe and keep up the good and great work that all of you are doing. THANK YOU.

—Pearline 'Jean' M.
Louisville, Kentucky

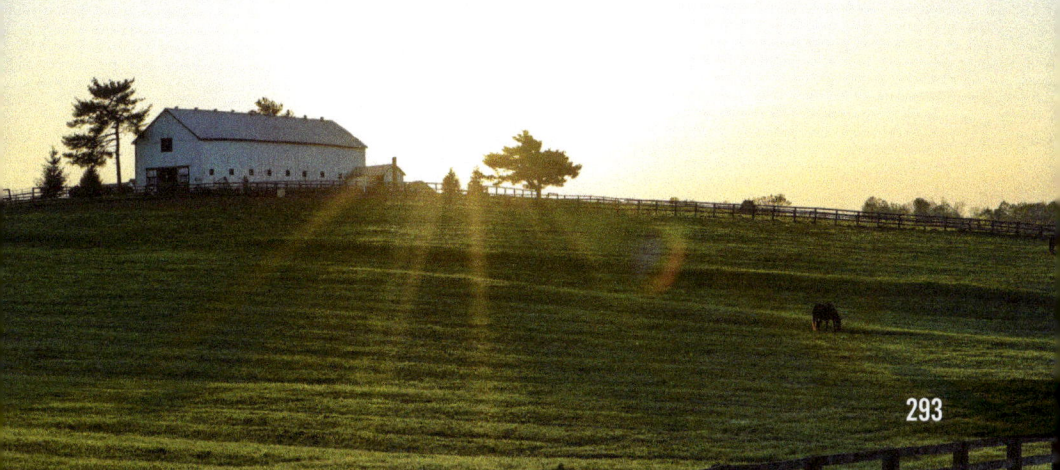

Let's R.E.S.T. CHECK POINT

You are through the Let's R.E.S.T. Morning Huddles.
This is a great time to STOP
and ASSESS how are you doing.

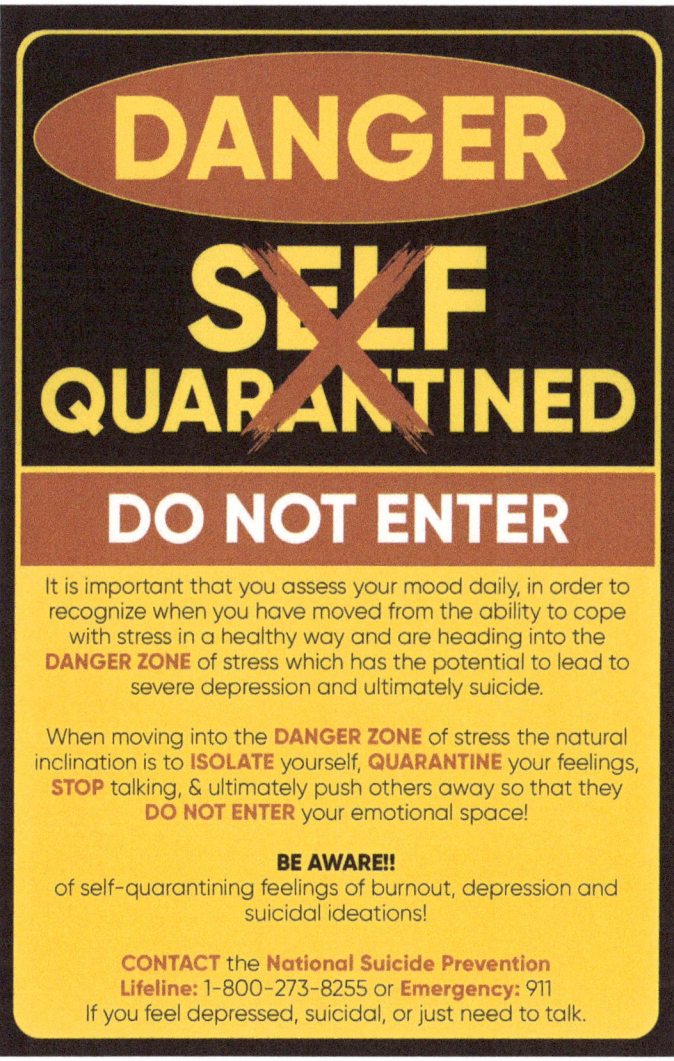

Throughout the remainder of this Let's R.E.S.T. Journal, continue to track your mood and assess whether you are heading into or have entered the DANGER Zone of stress & burnout!

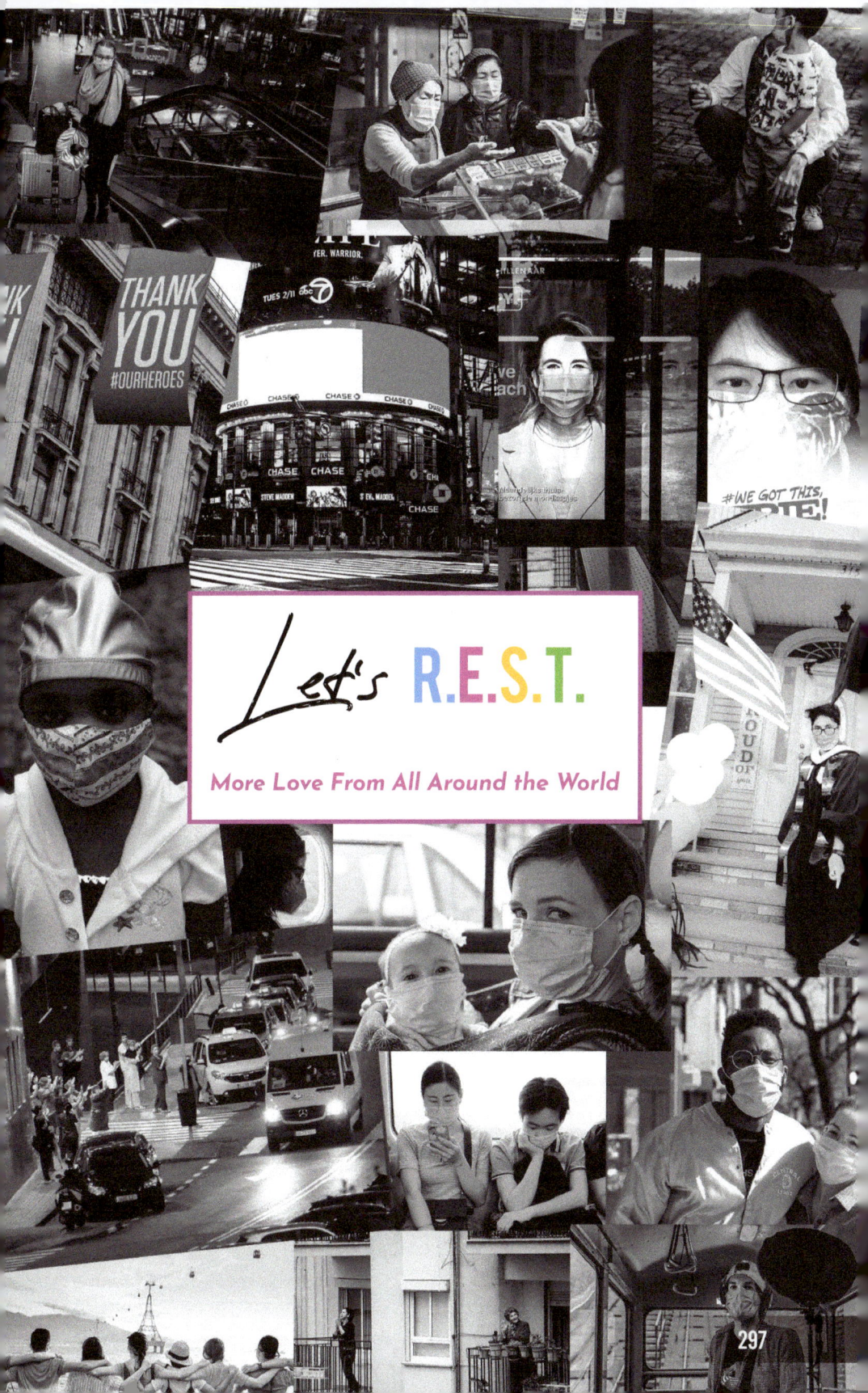

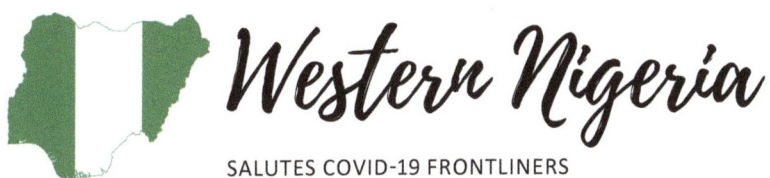

SALUTES COVID-19 FRONTLINERS

ORO IDUPE

Mo lo akokoyi lati dupe lowoOlorun fun iranlowoatiatilehin re niakokoajakalearun COVID-19 ni gbogbo agbaye.
Mo dupe lowoawononisegunti won un sisetakuntakun lati se itojuawon to lugbadiaisanyipelugbogboagbaraatiipa won, a moririise won niasiko yi; Olorunyoo fun won ni ere kikun.
OpolopoonisegunOyinbo lo ti padanuemi won, beeniopo ti ko aisanyi lo sile lo baawonebi won. Si awon to tiku, Olorunyoote won siafeferere, awon to lugbadiaisanyiOlorunyoo wo won San.
Mo rogbogboawononisegunoyinbokii won ma kare, ki won tesiwaju lati gboguntiaisan yii titi yoo fi kasenilepatapata, tialafia yoojobaniorileedeagbaye.

E se pupo, Olorunyoo ran yin lowo.
—Olufunke A.
Western Nigeria, Africa
(Yoruba language)

(English Translation):
WORD OF APPRECIATION

I am seizing this opportunity to thank God Almighty for His help and support since the breakout of this pandemic.
Also, I appreciate all frontliners and those working with them to take care of patients infected by COVID-19; God will reward you accordingly. I also remember those who lost their lives in the cause of caring for the patients and those who infected their loved ones. I pray the soul of the deceased will rest in perfect peace, and those who are down with the sickness will be healed by God's grace.
I am now appealing to all doctors and scientists in the universe not to relent in their efforts to fight COVID-19 until the world is healed of the pandemic and peace reigns all over the world.

Thank you, and God bless you all.

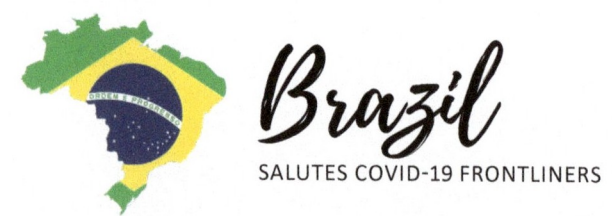

Brazil
SALUTES COVID-19 FRONTLINERS

The psalmist, in Psalm 1:1-2, declared, "Hear my cry, O God; attend unto my prayer. 2. From the end of the earth will I cry unto thee, when my heart is overwhelmed: lead me to the rock that is higher than I."

Being married to a physician, Bishop Terence Rhone, for more than thirty years has shown me how overwhelming the life of a health care worker can be. Most certainly, then, the COVID-19 crisis creates even greater stress levels for healthcare workers around the globe. Yet, there remains a Balm in Gilead who never leaves us nor forsakes us.

I pray that medical personnel everywhere will find solace in this fact as I pray earnestly for the Blood of Jesus to cover them and their families throughout this challenging time.

Prayerfully,
—First Lady Elizabeth Rhone,
Brazil

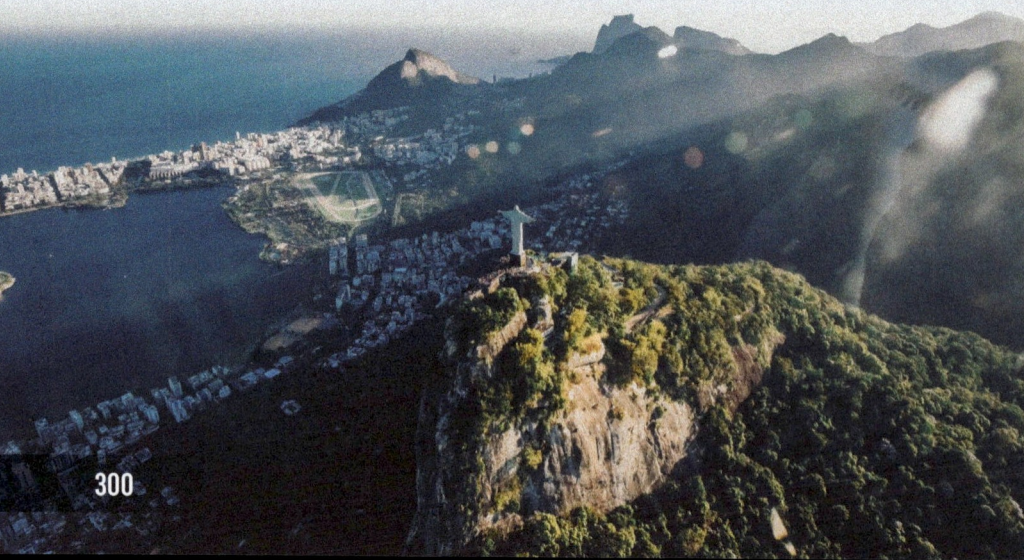

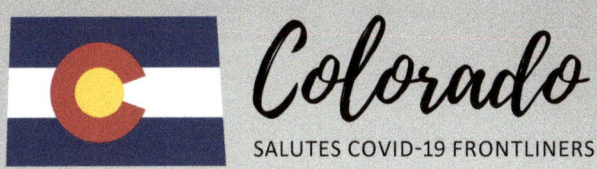

Colorado
SALUTES COVID-19 FRONTLINERS

*I am glad you are here. We never really appreciate those we really need until something like this hits us.
Keep fighting, but renew your inner spirit and remember you are not alone.*

—Matti B.
Denver, Colorado

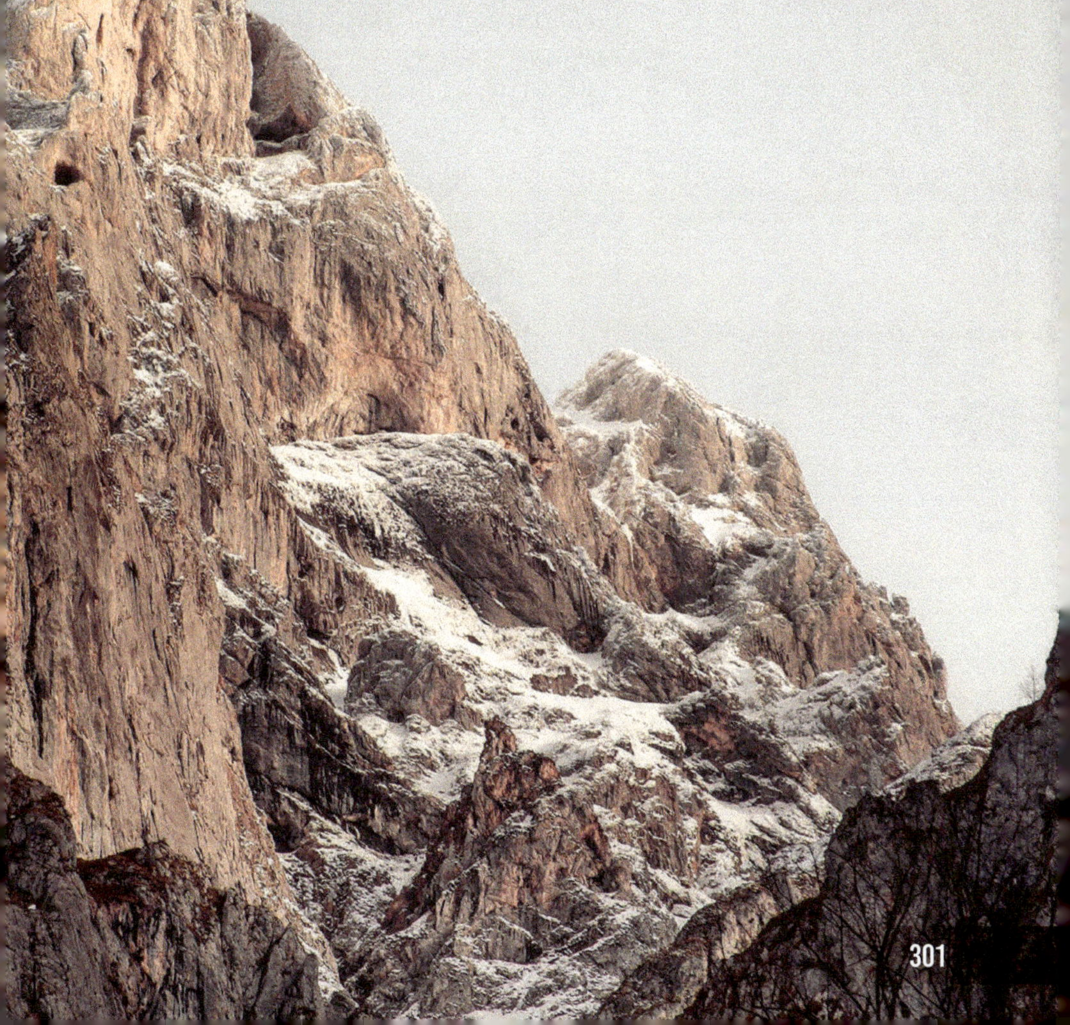

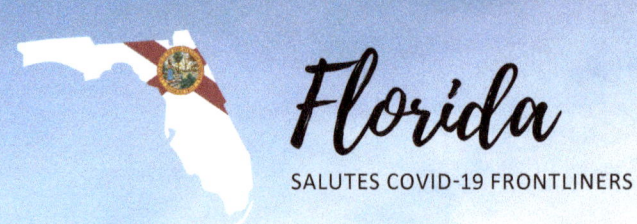

Florida
SALUTES COVID-19 FRONTLINERS

*Many are called, but only few are chosen.
You are the chosen ones.
We thank you for bravery, determination, and strength.
We support you in your fight against COVID-19.
You are all forever in our prayers.
We love you all. Stay safe.*

*—Shaquera A.
Orlando, Florida*

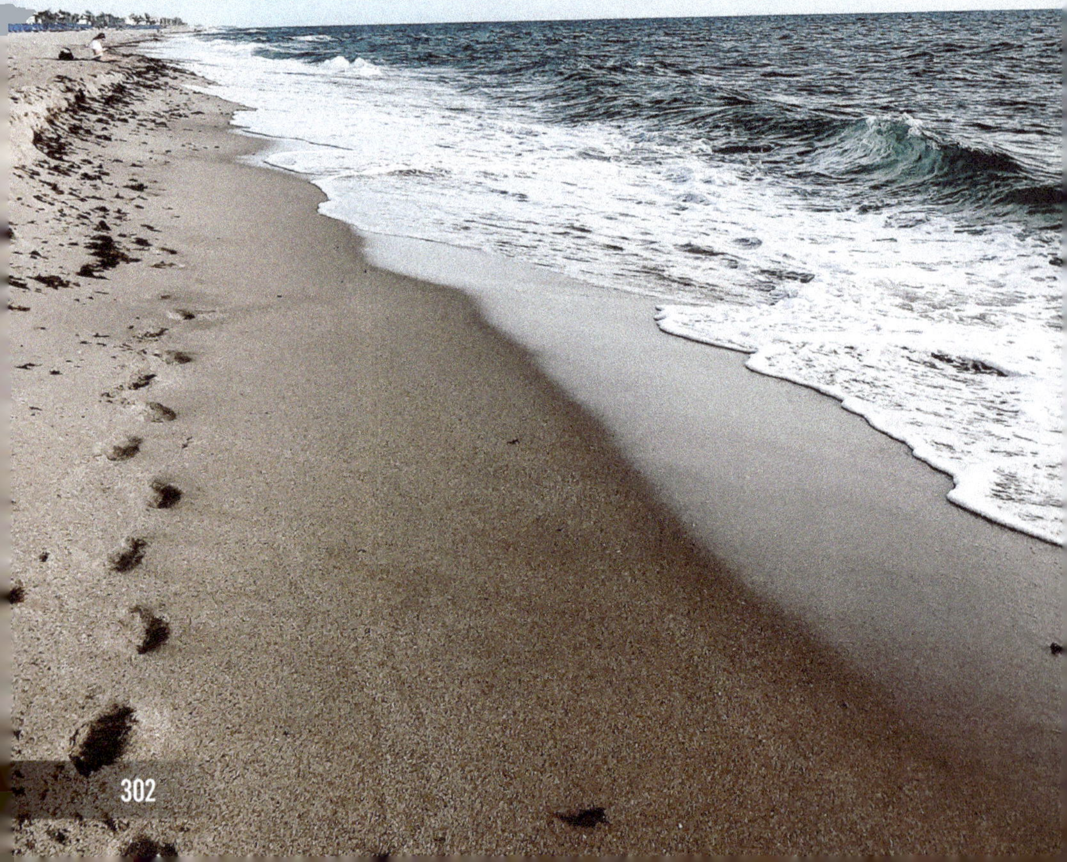

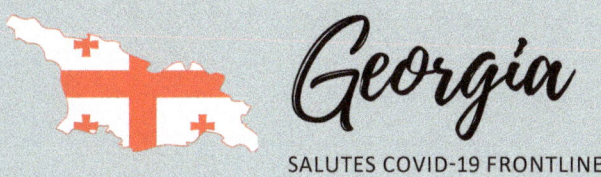

Georgia
SALUTES COVID-19 FRONTLINERS

My word of encouragement to Medical Front Liners of COVID-19 is mainly to show appreciation and to share a hearty thank-you for how many days and nights that medical teams serve in communities all over the world. From delivering babies to helping in the ICU, each job is very important and it is good to be able to commend all in uniform, and to reflect back on how much impact these Medical Front Liners of COVID-19 have made in the lives of others all over the world. Upon speaking one-on-one with a Medical Front Liner in the family it became more obvious as to how real their sacrifice is.

I've had an opportunity to talk to medical personnel and it made me want to devote more attention to praying for the COVID-19 medical frontliners especially during such an unprecedented time. It was beyond my human imagination to fathom what life must be like for them. Each day as pressures grow in the world, as a result of the pandemic, I think about medical frontliners having to multitask more than ever. With close relatives in need of care at local hospitals, it is important to keep encouraging medical personnel. As much as I had been complaining, it became a wake-up call to stop focusing on myself and remember to pray on behalf of the medical frontliners of COVID-19.

— Cassandra Y.
Atlanta, Georgia

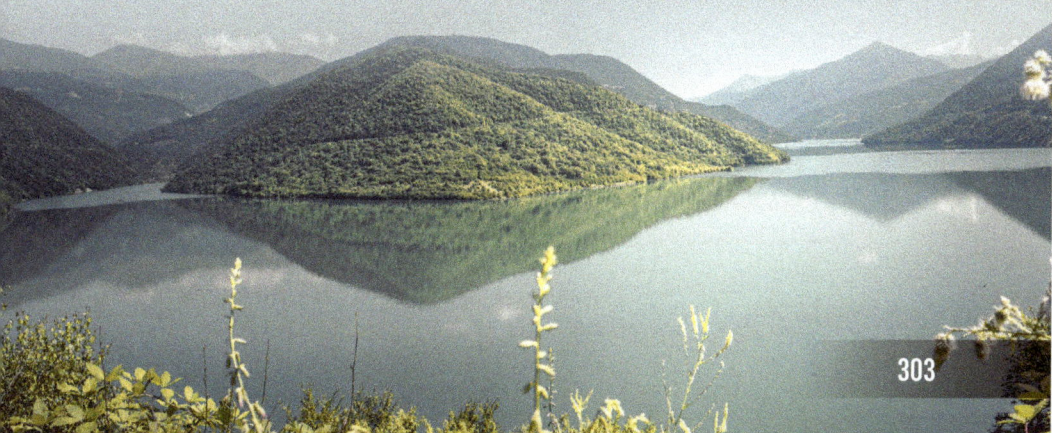

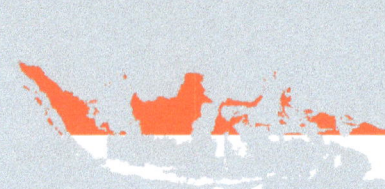

Indonesia

SALUTES COVID-19 FRONTLINERS

Versi Bahasa Indonesia:

Sejak pandemik mulai, sebagai penghubung pengungsi dan imigran di Kota Erie, saya mendengar berbagai macam cerita dari para pengungsi dan imigran terkait dengan virus corona. Mulai dari cerita seorang anak perempuan yang tidak bisa pulang ke negara asalnya (karena penerbangan internasional di tutup) ketika mendengar hasil tes ibunya positif hingga si ibu meninggal dunia; tiga generasi dalam keluarga yang seluruhnya terkena corona akibat tidak bisa menjaga jarak karena luas rumah yang relatif sempit; sampai dengan kendala bahasa untuk memahami bahaya COVID-19 itu sendiri.

Atas nama pengungsi dan imigran, perkenankan saya menyampaikan betapa kami sangat menghargai daya upaya para pekerja kesehatan, terutama yang berada di garis depan COVID-19. Terimakasih atas kepedulian bapak-ibu terhadap kesehatan kami. Kalian adalah pahlawan kesehatan!

—Niken Astari Carpenter
Erie, Pennsylvania, USA
Country of Origin: Republic of Indonesia

English version:

Since the outbreak started, as the New American Liaison of the City of Erie, I have heard many stories from refugees and immigrants in Erie related to coronavirus. The stories vary; from a daughter who couldn't go back to her homeland when hearing that her mother was tested positive for COVID-19 until the mother passed away; a three-generational family who all got COVID-19 due to the lack of space to adequately practice social distancing in their house; to the problem language barriers present to understanding the danger of COVID-19 itself.

Let me speak for the immigrant and refugee people of this country by saying your efforts are deeply valued and are essential to the well-being of these communities. So, for those of you on the frontline of COVID-19, please know that we appreciate what you do. You are HEROES!

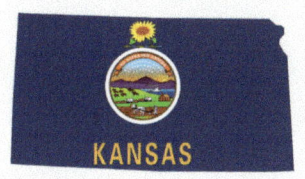

Kansas

SALUTES COVID-19 FRONTLINERS

Thank you to those caring for our communities. To all of the workers who have transformed their daily tasks from "routine medicine" to the focus on medicine surrounded by COVID-19, thank you. To the practice of medicine, caring for those who have become infected with COVID-19, we thank you. For the tireless effort you put forth to care for those who cross your path, we offer our greatest thanks. From the full clinic schedules (with more thrown on top) to hours outside of the clinic; and hospital shifts spent refreshing skills on intensive care (lest you should be called upon), you have given your patients another piece of your busy schedule. For those isolated from your families for weeks on end, after caring for a patient with COVID-19, and to those who gave up their very lives as a result of the privilege of caring for patients with COVID-19, we thank you. Praying God keeps you safe and encouraged as you do the task He has set before you. Well done!

—BD
Manhattan, Kansas

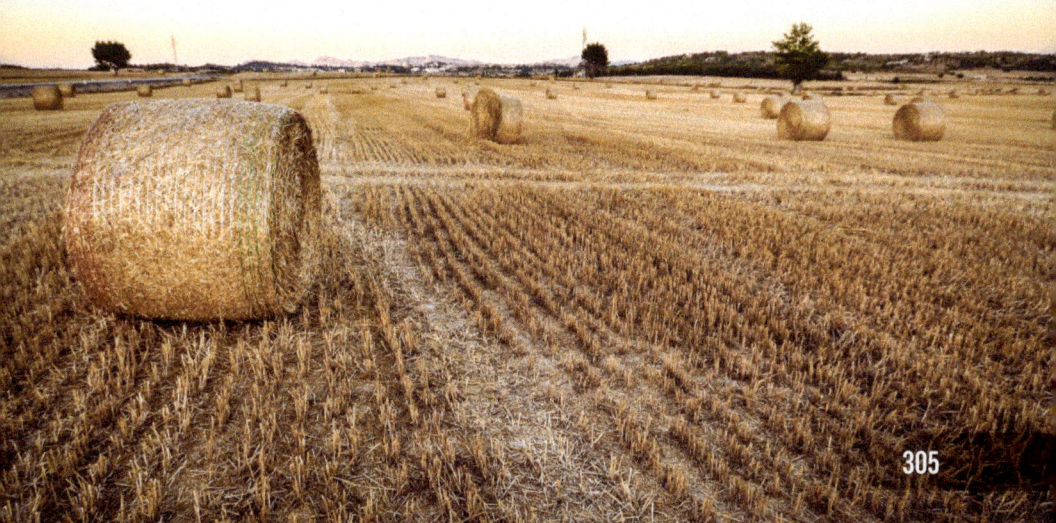

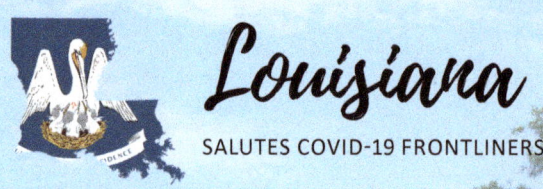

Louisiana
SALUTES COVID-19 FRONTLINERS

May God continue to lead and guide you into all truth and health: You are truly making a difference in the world, and you are surely impacting lives beyond your imagination. May God continue to encamp His angels of protection around you and your co-workers; and may you receive a 100-fold return on the love and help you seed into others' lives.

—Lovie H.
Mansfield, Louisiana

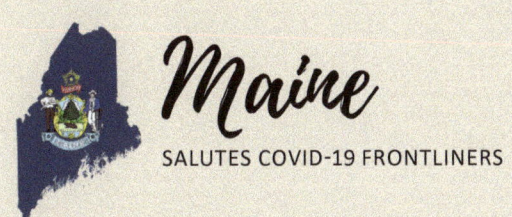
Maine
SALUTES COVID-19 FRONTLINERS

Never has the strength of nurses been seen more clearly. The ways we can adapt and overcome any obstacle thrown our way are unprecedented. We do it with love, humor, and compassion. I'm so proud to be a nurse and call these amazing people my colleagues.

*—Arienne H.
A nurse from Cape Elizabeth, Maine*

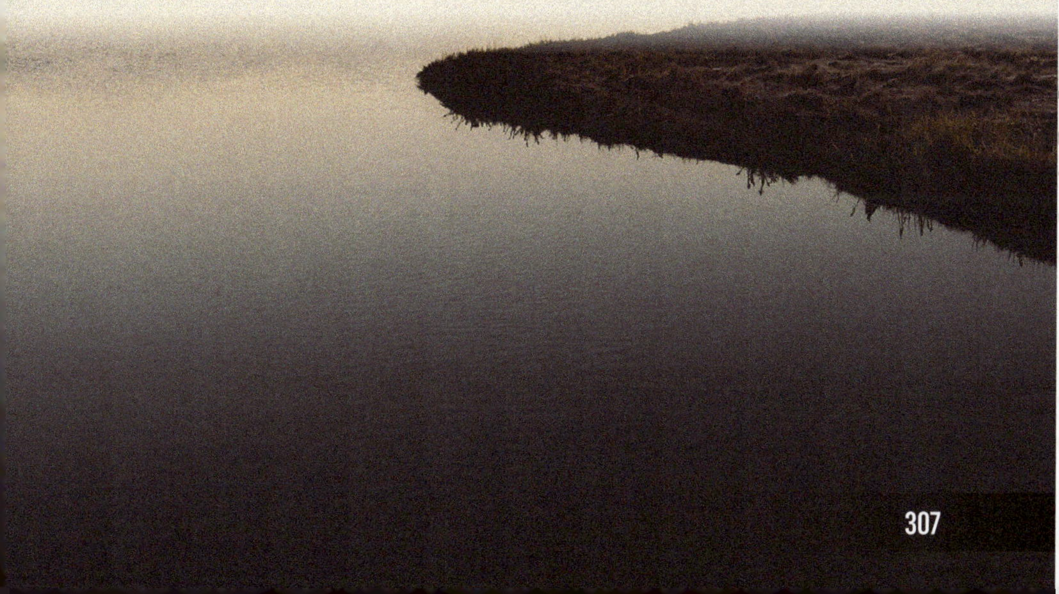

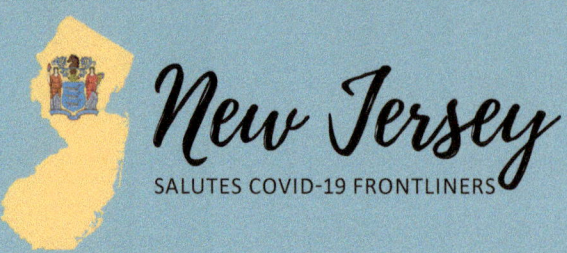

New Jersey
SALUTES COVID-19 FRONTLINERS

I have been in healthcare serving as a nurse for 17 years now. My reason for becoming a nurse was because I have a passion for wanting to care for others. Being there in the best of times and the worst of times, I can honestly say that as much as I've heard and learned about pandemics; I never thought that in my lifetime, I would be working in one such as now. However, I'm proud to say that I work with a great team; we have become closer than close. We are working long hours and are beyond exhaustion. We have included more music into our day. We have learned to laugh more and to share stories about how truly blessed we are. We've seen a lot of sorrow and pain, but we've learned to express our feelings amongst ourselves, which helps us deal with things better. Oh, by the way, did I forget to mention that we eat a lot of chocolate. Chocolate helps to alleviate stress. Many thanks to my fellow healthcare workers for the phenomenal job you do.

—Sandra T.
Ewing, New Jersey

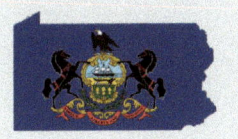

Pennsylvania

SALUTES COVID-19 FRONTLINERS

All frontline workers that stuck in there to help out and gave your all, I appreciate you. May God pour out His blessing on you and thank you for all you do. Love you guys!

—Patricia S.
Erie, Pennsylvania

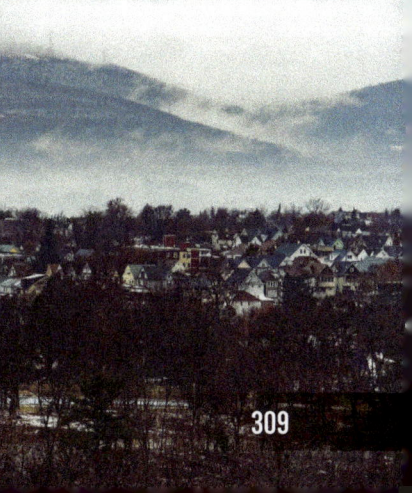

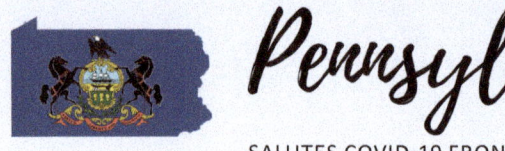

Pennsylvania

SALUTES COVID-19 FRONTLINERS

*You are needed,
You are important, and
You have my utmost respect!*

*—Trashawnda W.
Pittsburgh, Pennsylvania*

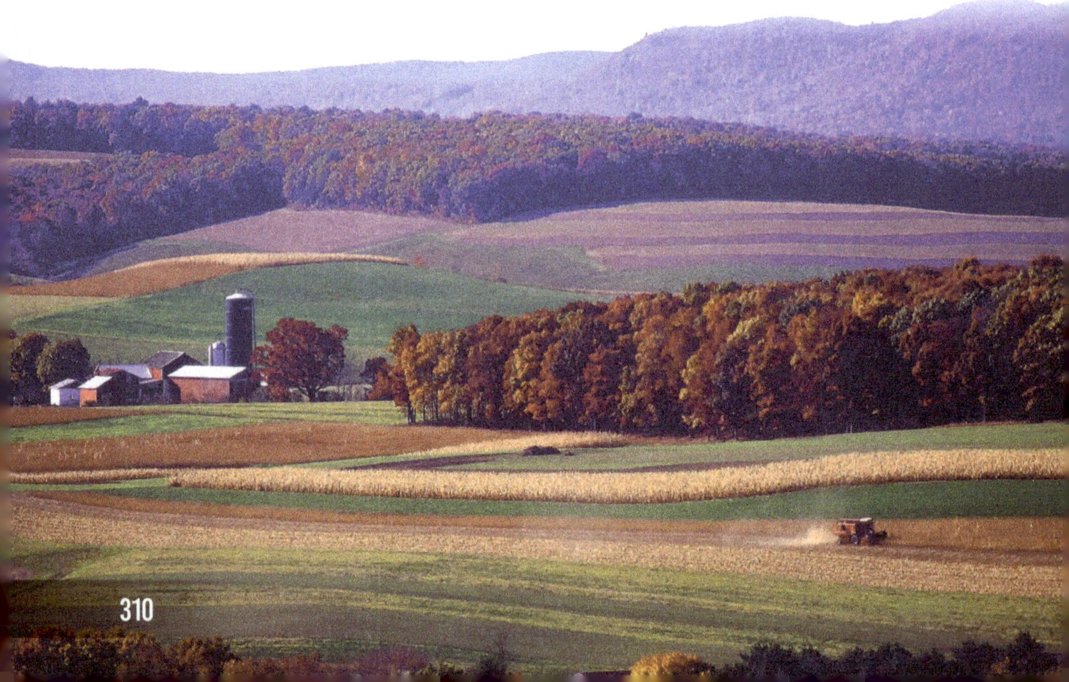

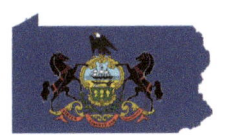

Pennsylvania

SALUTES COVID-19 FRONTLINERS

Blessings and hugs to each of you! I have witnessed the wisdom and care that you bring to your role and the heartfelt compassion that you give, beyond the job description. At a past hospital stay, I watched the caregiver lotion a patient's dry legs, gently move those legs for exercise and engage in conversation with a calm, joyful presence. I felt the love, even as a witness, and I was grateful. You bless us with your medical expertise and then allow that blessing to spill over abundantly with your time, passion, and belief in humanity. I see you giving your all during this pandemic, and I honor your leadership, Thanks.

*—Barbara J.
Pittsburgh, PA*

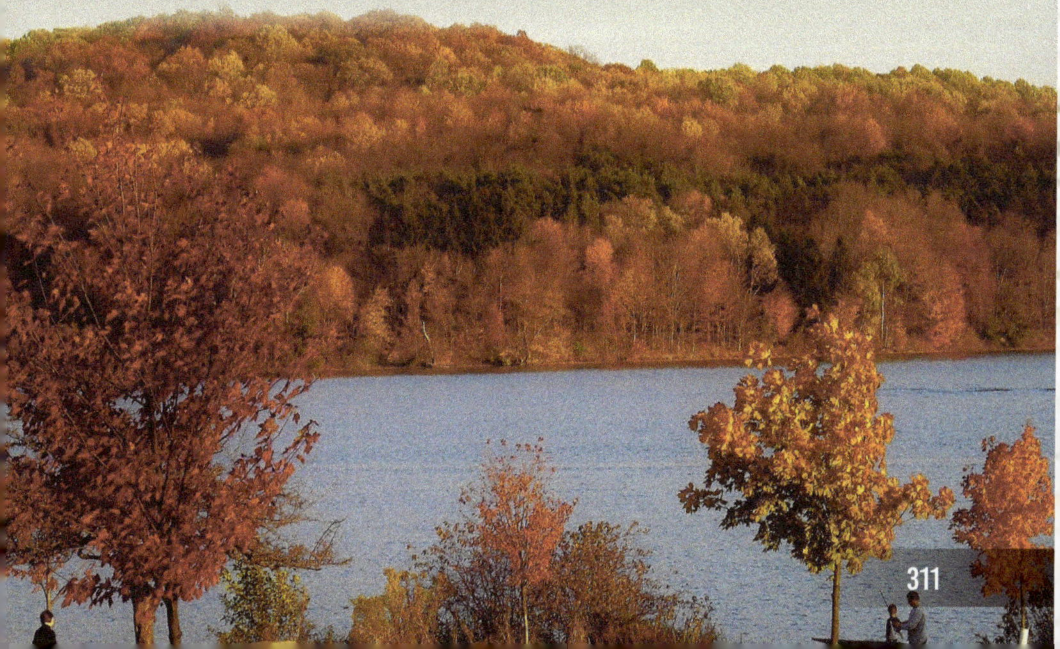

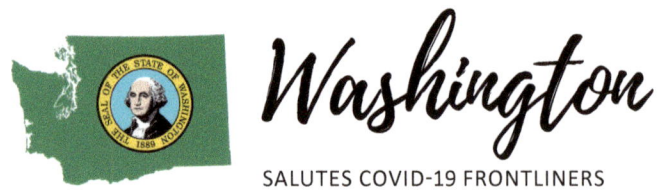

Washington

SALUTES COVID-19 FRONTLINERS

Hi! First of all, I want to thank the man upstairs for being there for all of us. May God continue to be the light in this maze that we are in right now.
Thank You Lord, for having your angels down here helping in the midst of the pandemic. We have people all around us that are willing to help us out -- the hospital is really being a blessing because they could just quit and let people fend for themselves, but no, they are gifted to help. May you shield everyone, Lord! Thank you to everyone in the world. May we be kind and help one another and show love to one another.

—Victoria T
Seattle, Washington

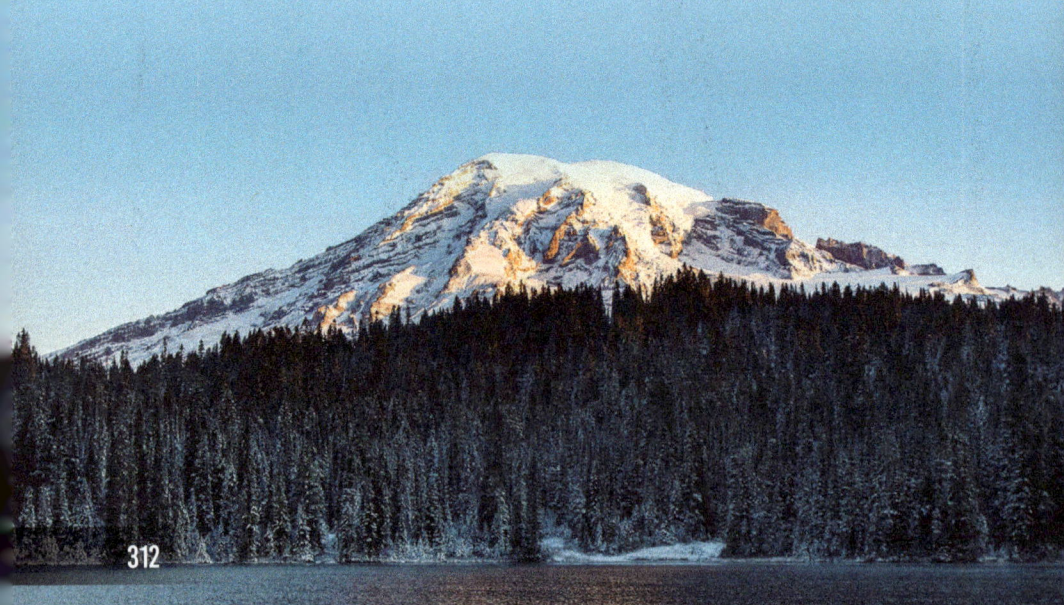

About the Author

Dr. Chevelta A. Smith is a board certified Obstetrician and Gynecologist and author of "Let's R.E.S.T. — Release Emotion and Stress Together: COVID-19 Frontliners Edition." Over the last five years, Dr. Chevelta has written both the "Can I Push?" book and journal in which she uniquely reveals to individuals through a dynamic medical-spiritual parallel, the importance of understanding the process to delivering their purpose. Within the last 18 years, she has touched the lives of many, via various ministry broadcasts, mentoring, coaching, and her previous radio talk show, Straight Talk with Dr. Chevelta. She is well known for her phenomenal teaching style and animated, yet powerful, public speaking. In her latest work, she provides a wonderful audio platform of daily messages to encourage fellow physicians who are working in this season of pandemic to Release Emotion and Stress Together (R.E.S.T.) with the goal of restoring their resilience and ultimately their strength to fulfill their purpose as medical professionals. Dr. Chevelta is a Navy veteran, who is now serving in Houston, Texas as a physician on the frontlines of this COVID-19 war. As a result, she not only understands what many medical professionals are feeling worldwide, but has personally experienced the associated fear and stress with working in this pandemic. Like many of her colleagues, she too has experienced the unavoidable exposure, during patient care, to this deadly virus. When she is not on the frontlines working, Dr. Chevelta loves bike riding (along the Bayou) with her husband, cooking, and good ole' family time.

www.ingramcontent.com/pod-product-compliance
Ingram Content Group UK Ltd.
Pitfield, Milton Keynes, MK11 3LW, UK
UKHW051557190426
11946UKWH00026B/130